Praise for *The Psychedelic Seeker's Guide*

"A foundational reference for the expanding psychedelic community of both providers and travelers. Whether for healing, psychological insight, or spiritual development, the kind of preparation Hunter describes is essential. With the expertise of an experienced traveler, she covers practical considerations, concerns for safety, and existential challenges. I imagine this book will be dog-eared, underlined, and shared for generations of psychedelic explorers. Read it carefully and stay safe!"

—RACHEL HARRIS, PhD, author of *Listening to Ayahuasca* and *Swimming in the Sacred*

"In an era enthralled by the therapeutic promise of psychedelics, the labyrinth of information, considerations, and potential choices for the seeker remains as intricate as it is understated. Like Ariadne's guiding thread, Kristina Hunter's expert yet accessible voice gently unspools a path of clarity and discernment for those contemplating a psychedelic journey. A much-needed contribution to this unfolding field."

—SUSANA BUSTOS, PhD, author of *The Shamanic Odyssey*

"Drawing on extensive experience in guiding, teaching, and integration—as well as the author's own healing journey—*The Psychedelic Seeker's Guide* emphasizes discernment, ethical relationship, and thoughtful preparation. Readers learn how to choose a trustworthy facilitator, understand the differences among medicines, and integrate powerful experiences responsibly. This is a grounded and reassuring companion for anyone considering or returning to ceremony."

—KYLEA TAYLOR, LMFT, founder of InnerEthics and author of *The Ethics of Caring*

"This book is a lucid and trustworthy guide for anyone considering psychedelic work—seekers, trainees, and seasoned facilitators alike. With poetic clarity and ethical rigor, Hunter offers practical frameworks for reducing risk, maximizing benefit, and discerning the right guide, setting, and medicine. Her candid discussion of both promise and peril—including warning signs of harmful facilitation—equips readers to engage this terrain with wisdom and care. This is an essential resource for informed, responsible psychedelic practice."

—JASON BUTLER, PhD, author of *Integral Psychedelic Therapy*

"We are coming out of over half a century of radical, misguided government suppression of medicines that would benefit millions of people. In this new phase of slightly less suppression, well over 95 percent of the administration of these medicines remains underground with neither rules nor regulations nor controls on the purity of the substances being administered. Kristina Hunter's book is extremely valuable, as it provides us with details on responsible use. Read *The Psychedelic Seeker's Guide* and keep it in your library as a ready reference."

—DR. RICHARD LOUIS MILLER, author and host of the *Mind Body Health & Politics* radio broadcast

"Real, empowering, and down to earth: Those are the words that come to mind while reading *The Psychedelic Seeker's Guide*. True to her personal integrity, intellectual precision, and lived experience, Kristina Hunter transfers the power of the psychedelic journey from the guide to the seeker. . . . I hope everyone considering psychedelics reads this book to enter the space with eyes wide open."

—SERGIO RODRIGUEZ-CASTILLO, LMFT, PhD, author of "An Integral Blueprint for Psychedelic-Assisted Therapy"

"A vital and refreshing perspective on the nuances of power, projection, ethics, and agency for people seeking to enter into the psychedelic realm, perhaps for the first time. . . . In a world of psychedelic charlatans new to the medicine whose only credential is a weekend workshop, Kristina Hunter has earned every drop of wisdom presented here. She is the real deal."

—SIMON YUGLER, psychedelic therapist and author of *Psychedelics and the Soul*

"*The Psychedelic Seeker's Guide* brings a breath of fresh air. . . . The information shared in this book will be immensely helpful to seekers for self-advocacy in communication with guides, enhanced benefits, and fostering safety. I highly recommend this book to anyone involved in psychedelic healing—and especially to seekers—for its valuable perspective and practical wisdom."

—DR. CEDAR BARSTOW, author of *Right Use of Power* and founder of the Right Use of Power Institute

"With over forty years of experience as a nurse practitioner in psychiatry, forensic sexual assault, and addiction medicine, I see *The Psychedelic Seeker's Guide* as an essential primer. . . . This book's relevance to the recovery community is especially notable. Even after achieving abstinence, many find themselves feeling constrained or stuck. The familiar guidance to 'do more step work' or 'turn it over' may offer limited relief and, at times, deepen frustration and hopelessness. For some individuals, carefully supported engagement with psychedelics may offer a different pathway—one that facilitates deeper insight, emotional release, and movement toward self-acceptance. I would confidently recommend this book to both professionals and individuals seeking informed guidance. It is a clear, practical, and timely contribution to the field."

—LUCRETIA BOLIN, PhD, APRN-BC

"*The Psychedelic Seeker's Guide* weaves Hunter's personal experiences as a practitioner, educator, and student of psychedelic medicine. Hunter does not shy away from taboo topics and empowers the reader to ask difficult questions. I highly recommend her book for individuals seeking grounded, wise, and direct guidance. In times of AI, it's more and more important to hear from folks on the ground, deeply connected to community, and willing to speak truth to power."

—MARY SANDERS, LCSW, politicized therapist, educator, and community builder

"Kristina Hunter's *The Psychedelic Seeker's Guide* is clearly presented, thoughtfully worded, and drawn from her decades of experience as a seeker and a survivor of life challenges. . . . In a world where psychedelic seekers must find their way through a mysterious forest of possible choices, this book is a clear and helpful trail map."

—KATHLEEN HARRISON, independent scholar and ethnobotanist and president and cofounder of Botanical Dimensions

THE PSYCHEDELIC SEEKER'S GUIDE

THE PSYCHEDELIC SEEKER'S GUIDE

How to Prepare Wisely, Journey Safely, and Find Your Medicine

KRISTINA HUNTER

North Atlantic Books
Huichin, unceded Ohlone land
Berkeley, California

North Atlantic Books
An educational nonprofit organization
Huichin, unceded Ohlone land
2526 Martin Luther King Jr Way
Berkeley, CA 94704 USA
www.northatlanticbooks.com

Cover photos © JPC-PROD, Md Amir Hossain, anmbph via Getty Images and Dr_Microbe via Adobe Stock
Cover design by Jasmine Hromjak
Book design by Happenstance Type-O-Rama

Acquisitions editor: Francesca Walker • Production editor: Janelle Ludowise
Copyeditor: Christopher Church • Proofreader: Chuck Hutchinson
Indexer: Tim Tate

North Atlantic Books's publications are distributed to the US trade and internationally by Penguin Random House Publisher Services. For further information, visit our website at www.northatlanticbooks.com.

The authorized representative in the EU for product safety and compliance is Eucomply OÜ, Pärnu mnt 139b-14, 11317 Tallinn, Estonia, hello@eucompliancepartner.com, +33757690241.

DISCLAIMER: The following information is intended for general information purposes only. The publisher does not advocate illegal activities but does believe in the right of individuals to have free access to information and ideas. Any application of the material set forth in the following pages is at the reader's discretion and is their sole responsibility.

Library of Congress Cataloging-in-Publication data is available from the publisher upon request.

ISBN: 979-8-88984-311-5 (paperback)
ISBN: 979-8-88984-312-2 (ebook)

1 2 3 4 5 6 7 8 9 KPC 31 30 29 28 27 26

Printed in the United States of America

Dedicated to those who faithfully tend the mysteries—
whether celebrated or forbidden.

Contents

Preface

At the age of twenty-eight, a week before I was to start graduate school in psychology, I found myself sitting in a hospital bed. I had been experiencing mysterious pain, fatigue, and weight loss for three months. Despite multiple doctor visits and tests, no one could tell me what was wrong. For the second time that month, I drove myself to the emergency room with excruciating abdominal pain. Finally, after a battery of scans, I got answers. An older doctor sat down across from me and, with a pained look, told me I had a large tumor growing inside me. "Endometrial adenocarcinoma," she said. "Uterine cancer." I had four days to prepare for extensive surgery to remove multiple organs and lymph nodes. I was in shock, but relieved to have a diagnosis.

A few days after my surgery, I was still floating in a morphine-induced dream state when the head surgeon walked into my room. He stood at the foot of my hospital bed, clipboard in hand, and told me matter-of-factly, "The cancer has spread. It's stage four, and you'll need aggressive chemotherapy. Plan to start in six weeks."

I nodded. After he left the room, I wondered, "What the hell *is* chemotherapy anyway?" I knew it made people lose their hair and throw up. But was it pills? Did it go into your veins? I grabbed my phone and looked it up. Besides a few rounds of antibiotics, I had had little contact with conventional medicine at that point. My mom, who had apprenticed as a midwife before becoming a nurse, leaned toward alternative healing. After conventional medicines had failed to treat my chronic ear infections and high fevers at age five, a homeopathic remedy healed them. Years later, my recurrent strep throat infections disappeared after taking herbs prescribed by a Chinese herbalist.

A month later, I met the oncologist assigned to my case. It was early November, and the winter chill had just set in. After thirty minutes reviewing my chart, the doctor named the drugs that would be in my chemotherapy cocktail. I recognized the name of the primary one from my extensive online research and interrupted, "Doesn't that one cause long-term heart damage?"

She stopped and looked at me for a long moment. "Yes, there is a risk of heart damage after the ten-year mark. But Ms. Hunter," she took a deep breath and lowered her voice, "you'll be lucky to be here in ten years." Statistically speaking, even with the strongest drugs, my chance of survival after five years would only be 15 percent.

Fifteen percent. There was a high likelihood I was going to die before age thirty-five. Not only did I need to navigate a complex medical situation, but I was facing psychological territory for which I had few tools. I sought a second opinion and weighed my options. Although it went against the advice of my oncologist, I negotiated for a different combination of drugs with less severe long-term side effects. I also wove in herbal medicine, acupuncture, and daily cannabis, a benevolent plant medicine that revived my appetite and helped me sleep through the night. I was fortunate. Today, I remain cancer-free, or as my doctors say, "in remission." Conventional medicine—with its scans, plastic tubes, and manufactured chemicals—helped save my life. However, conventional medicine wasn't able to help me put myself back together in the aftermath of its effects.

After my treatment concluded and my scans were clear, I felt physically depleted, emotionally hollowed out, and anxious about recurrence. I knew that following an anticancer diet, exercising, and doing daily qigong would give me the best chance of staying healthy. But how could I do it all while, at the deepest level, I was wrestling with existential questions, like: How do I live in this scarred body now missing vital organs? How should I spend my days not knowing how many I have left? Will I live to see forty? What I needed was medicine for my soul. Luckily, I knew where to find it.

By then, I had been working with psychedelics for fifteen years. As a teenager, I had the good fortune of eating my first handful of psilocybin mushrooms in the woods of California. At the time, my inner world had felt dark and rigid. I was unknowingly living with PTSD as a result of an encounter with gun violence at the age of ten and the challenges of day-to-day reality in a family struggling with depression and alcoholism. On eating those humble-looking brown mushrooms, life suddenly appeared magical and full of possibilities. I laughed again, feeling suddenly lighter, remembering who I was beneath the fear and anger. I recognized that these mushrooms—and the other psychedelic medicines I immediately sought out—were extraordinary.

At twenty, my growing interest in the inner dimensions that plant medicines revealed and the joy they sparked in me drew me to Iquitos, Peru. This was 2003, just before the ayahuasca tourism boom, and I asked around for a week before I found a guide who would take me deeper into the rainforest to experience a ceremony. I was eager to meet traditional practitioners who prepared and served these medicines with care and respect. During this and subsequent trips to Central and South America, I attended ayahuasca, *huachuma* (San Pedro) cactus, and psilocybin mushroom ceremonies with Indigenous *curanderos,* mestizo healers, and religious communities. I encountered diverse cosmologies and approaches to healing, all rooted in reverence for these sacred medicines and the earth they come from.

Back in the States, I began attending festivals and volunteering in psychedelic harm reduction tents. I met psychedelic guides working in styles that blended traditional healing with psychological frameworks. I began assisting with group ayahuasca ceremonies in California alongside a facilitator who had apprenticed with traditional healers in the Amazon. Like many, I became increasingly enchanted by the cross-cultural practices of ceremonial prayer and song, plant sacraments, and human conviviality. My love affair with the community that formed around these ceremonies and the inner landscapes they revealed—a world that seemed far more compelling than mainstream culture—became a central force in my life.

I also continued to encounter the misinformation and moral panic that permeated attitudes about psychedelics as well as the extreme inequity in access to them. I figured the best way for me to contribute was to become a therapist so I could do this work directly with people. I enrolled in graduate school, hoping to join the first legal wave of psychedelic therapists offering MDMA therapy, and maybe one day, psilocybin.

It was then, one week before I was to start a graduate program, that I received my cancer diagnosis. To address the enormous existential questions that it awakened, I returned to psychedelic medicine. This time, however, I didn't come for exploration; I came for healing. I returned to ayahuasca ceremonies and participated in guided journeys with MDMA and psilocybin mushrooms. I purged out the anesthesia, chemotherapy, and countless other drugs that had been infused and injected into me for survival. I shook the fear out of my system, feeling the fibers in my wounded tissues reweave themselves. I prayed for guidance and saw into the inherited familial patterns I needed to confront to rebuild my strength, all while being reminded that life is cocreative and mysterious. Perhaps the most healing gift I received was a vision of myself in the future—alive. The belief that I probably wouldn't make it more than five years began to dissolve, and my psychedelic journeys helped me open my heart, reminding me I wasn't the only one suffering. "Why me?" turned into "Why not me?" I found my footing again. These medicines proved themselves as allies I could trust: confrontational at times, yet fiercely compassionate. I was humbled.

I attempted to return to graduate school three times, but because of long-term side effects from my cancer treatment, I wasn't able to finish my studies. Eventually I accepted that I had a different path to walk—one centered on personal experience and apprenticeship rather than formal education. I studied alternative approaches to counseling, continued to assist ayahuasca ceremonies, and eventually trained as a psychedelic guide. I wanted to offer others what I had been given: access to these life-changing medicines.

I started offering psychedelic integration support and eventually began to accompany others on psychedelic journeys. I also cowrote a book on healing through expanded states of consciousness, which was published in 2019. Doing so was an opportunity to spend hours with an older practitioner who had been exploring this terrain decades longer than I had. I thought I was beginning to understand the territory. I thought I was learning what good work looked like.

In the same year, I began hearing troubling stories from clinical trials and ceremonial settings: tales of facilitators initiating sexual relationships with participants during or immediately after sessions, in the United States and abroad. Then, in 2021, multiple allegations of sexual misconduct surfaced against a well-known psychedelic guide and trainer in a community I had been close to for years. The abuse occurred while their clients were in vulnerable altered states of consciousness.

Learning that serious harm was happening behind closed doors—doors meant to protect sacred healing work—was devastating. I listened to the survivors, sought supervision, and spent time with elders and psychedelic guides from other communities. Ultimately I severed contact with those who minimized, rationalized, or justified the abuse.

As people from other communities shared similar stories, a clear pattern emerged: inappropriate relationships initiated by facilitators, manipulative power dynamics, and therapeutic work that caused harm. This was happening alongside genuine ethical healing, but the scope of the problem was undeniable. I considered walking away from psychedelic work entirely, but I still believed in the potential of these medicines. If people were getting hurt by facilitators this often, perhaps facilitator training was the place to focus.

When I was hired to help create a Psychedelic Facilitation Certificate Program at the University of California, Berkeley, I saw it as exactly the opportunity I'd been looking for. I helped develop the curriculum and was part of the instructional team for three years, during which I focused on two areas: supervising the ethics curriculum with Kylea Taylor, a therapist specializing in ethics and expanded states, and overseeing practicum training that would prepare graduates to become licensed psilocybin facilitators in Oregon. Over three years, we trained 110 professionals—doctors, nurses, therapists, clergy, and traditional medicine lineage holders from diverse cultural, racial, and gender backgrounds, many of whom now offer legal psychedelic care across the country and abroad.

Through this work I came to see a gap that training facilitators alone couldn't address. I kept thinking back to my cancer treatment and the survivors I'd met since. What many of us had in common was that we refused to be passive recipients of care. We researched our diagnoses, questioned our doctors, and insisted on understanding every treatment and medication going into our bodies. We became what's sometimes called "expert" patients—demanding, perhaps harder to work with, but damn determined to survive. While it's fairly easy to find information about cancer treatment, it's much harder to find clear guidance about psychedelic work, which means people enter these experiences without knowing what to look for or what questions to ask. An imbalance of power already exists in these relationships, and it is further amplified when seekers don't understand what they're getting themselves into. Those seeking psychedelic healing need their own foundation of knowledge to navigate this territory safely.

Surviving cancer required that I become an active agent in my own recovery by asking hard questions, making informed choices, and deciding when to trust experts and when to trust myself. The path of psychedelic healing demands the same active participation. I wrote this book to support that participation. I'm sharing the guidance I've gathered over the years: both what can support your deepest healing and what can go wrong. My hope is that this knowledge helps you move forward with clarity and confidence, whatever path you choose.

Introduction

The police officers passed glossy photos of drugs around my fifth-grade classroom. They were there for our weekly Drug Abuse Resistance Education (DARE) session, explaining the dangers of drugs while encouraging us to report any use at home. According to them, all drugs were equally destructive. They showed us the photos accompanied by a description of each substance's effects. Marijuana, the description said, could cause "changes in the sense of space and time." Well, that caught my attention.

I had been around drugs enough to know the truth was more complex than what they described. These were powerful substances, but I knew they were all quite different. I knew people smoked marijuana without becoming addicted, as the police insisted they would. The actual effect those DARE meetings had on me and many other kids was not the intended one. I became even more curious about drugs. Three years later, while browsing through a family friend's overflowing bookshelf, I found *The Psychedelic Experience*, written by Harvard researchers in the early 1960s.[1] This radical book reimagined a thousand-year-old Tibetan manual for navigating the dying process as a map for psychedelic journeys. I took it home and secretly read it cover to cover.

Twenty-five years later, I sat next to a woman as she recalled the cruel words her mom had been telling her since she was a toddler, and it crushed my heart. Maria, a teacher in her forties, had survived years of neglect and emotional abuse from her deceased mother. Now, at the height of a psilocybin mushroom journey, her cheeks wet with tears, she asked out loud how anyone could say these things to another human, let alone their own daughter. I had no response. Her mother's behavior was beyond my comprehension. But about three hours into her journey, Maria sat up. "She was envious of my innocence. She didn't know how to be a mother, and she was overwhelmed." Her hands went to her heart as she continued giving voice to her insights. "I don't need to carry this with me anymore. I'm ready to let her go and live my life. Something larger is holding me now—and it's time to let it in."

After her journey, Maria said she felt unburdened. She didn't excuse her mother's abuse, but she saw a bigger picture. She said it was as though she had felt her mother's confusion on a visceral level. The cruelty had never been about her; she'd done nothing wrong. She was done centering her life around that painful story and ready to move forward. Maria's shift came after years of therapy, but it was the support of the mushrooms that day that finally helped her take the next step. She was able to have that session with me because she was willing to take the legal risk; psilocybin remains prohibited in most US states.

Maria's story isn't unique. Thousands of people are discovering similar healing through psychedelic substances. And slowly the mainstream is catching up. Today, these once stigmatized medicines are steadily moving from the underground out into the light. Around the world, laws are shifting: Indigenous protections in Peru and Mexico, medical pathways in Australia and Canada, decriminalization in Portugal and the Czech Republic, and state-by-state legalization in the United States. Decades of prohibition driven by the US war on drugs—racist policies now widely recognized as a catastrophic failure—are slowly giving way to humane laws and increased access. Promising research is mounting as more universities and biotechnology companies study the therapeutic potential of many of these substances. It should be recognized that for millennia, many cultures have maintained unbroken relationships with plant medicines and clear guidance for their use, despite the violent attempts of colonialism to eradicate their traditions. But for many of us in the Global North who were raised outside these traditions, straightforward guidance on navigating psychedelic healing safely is hard to find.

I've written this book to guide you through the multifaceted landscape of psychedelic healing so you can navigate it with greater personal agency. I define agency as the power to think for yourself and shape your experience through your own choices and actions. I address both the benefits and the risks of these medicines, helping you clarify your intentions and weigh your options.

In my years of working with people seeking psychedelic experiences, I've encountered the full range of motivations. Some come with curiosity, seeking a fresh perspective, clarity about their life direction, or spiritual communion. Others sense something missing after achieving the material successes in life, wondering, "Is this all there is?" Still others come with years of struggle behind them: chronic illness, decades-old anger, generational addiction, or symptoms of trauma that conventional approaches haven't been able to resolve. When they look at their options, psychedelics stand out, whether as a path to deeper understanding or as a last resort.

Seekers of healing deserve protection, care, and guidance. Fortunately, there are many well-trained psychedelic guides and professionally run clinics to be found. But there are also therapists, coaches, and bodyworkers who complete a weekend workshop and begin offering their services as psychedelic guides without understanding how much more training is needed. And worse, some people who call themselves guides use psychedelics and spiritual language to justify harmful behavior. How can you tell the difference?

Whether you're exploring legal options or navigating unregulated terrain, it's up to you to be as informed as possible, to ask the right questions, and to decide where to place your trust. You are the authority on your experience, even in a supportive setting with a skilled facilitator. Learning to make informed decisions, set boundaries, and trust yourself is central to healing.

If you take only one thing from this introduction, let it be this: A psychedelic journey is a rare opportunity to meet yourself at a depth most people never access. This opportunity deserves your full attention, your time, and your respect. It also deserves the utmost care and respect from anyone you invite to sit by your side while you are wide open and vulnerable. They should keep you safe and never ask you to surrender your critical thinking.

Is This Book for You?

If you are considering a psychedelic experience and want to learn more so you can engage with discernment, this book is for you. It will answer questions like: What are the risks involved? What setting would best support me? Should I work with a psychedelic guide, and if so, how will I know if they're trustworthy? What does intentional preparation and thoughtful integration look like? How can I move beyond a fleeting experience and create real change in my life?

This book is not a manual for self-guided high-dose journeys. I don't recommend that approach, especially for beginners. However, I do include guidance for those who choose to explore psychedelics without a facilitator because I know many people don't have access to a guide, can't afford one, or prefer not to pursue guided work. Many people choose to journey in community or with friends, so I offer suggestions to help make that approach safer and more supportive.

Nor is this book a comprehensive encyclopedia of every psychoactive medicine or a manifesto about what is wrong with the psychedelic renaissance. I'm not here to sell you anything. What I am here to do is to help you approach one of the most powerful experiences available to a human being with the seriousness it deserves. If you choose not to use psychedelics, that's okay with me. However, *should* you decide to explore, I want you to have the information to do so safely with an appropriate understanding of their power, risks, and limitations. After reading this book, you'll have a clearer sense of whether this path is right for you and, if so, what steps to take next.

Based on my years of experience, I've come to believe psychedelics are most transformative when set within a larger framework of preparation and integration with the support of a guide or group facilitator. However, community-based and peer support models can also be effective. Regardless of the setting, integration—bringing insights from expanded states into daily life—is essential for lasting change, and a healthy relationship with any powerful medicine hinges on authentic humility and cultivated respect.

This book is organized to walk you through the entire journey, helping you approach each step with care. The first section gives you foundational knowledge: understanding how psychedelics catalyze healing and assessing your safety and readiness. The next section helps you make key decisions: choosing your setting, deciding whether to work with a guide, and understanding the powers and limitations of different medicines. The core of the book guides you through the arc of the experience itself: preparing intentionally, crafting an intention worthy of the opportunity, navigating the journey with courage and openness, and integrating your insights so they take root in your life. The final section addresses the shadow side: how to navigate complex dynamics with guides, and how to recognize red flags and respond to abuse.

Throughout, I place a strong emphasis on working with guides. Psychedelics make you vulnerable; they lower your psychological defenses and can temporarily render you physically incapacitated. This makes the presence of a skilled guide invaluable and healing more accessible, but also makes harm more possible. Most people have no framework for recognizing unethical behavior until it's too late. When you're this vulnerable, you need to know exactly who you're with beforehand, not after something goes wrong. And even if you don't work with a guide, the information in these chapters can still help you. It applies equally to working with a therapist, coach, or spiritual teacher.

Where I'm Coming From

This book does not cover every medicine or cultural tradition of psychedelic healing. I focus on what I know. I have years of counseling training but I'm not a licensed therapist. I have worked in academia but I am not an academic. I've had the good fortune to spend time with Indigenous and mestizo teachers who carry healing lineages passed down through generations, but I do not claim any one lineage as my own. For their legal protection, I have chosen not to name my teachers. I speak from my experience as a white woman with primarily European roots living in the United States.

I began exploring psychedelics early and continue to use them, despite their prohibition, with minimal fear of consequences because of my skin color and socioeconomic status. The economic barriers, social impacts, and legal risks of engaging with psychedelics or any prohibited substance are unequally distributed, and the psychedelic field remains predominantly white and financially inaccessible. These are systemic issues beyond the scope of this book, yet they are critical to any honest discussion of psychedelic access and central to creating a more equitable field.

A Note on Language

Psychedelic medicines are more than just molecules or psychological tools. They are keys that reconnect us to the living magic of the cosmos. Many reverential terms exist for them, including *sacraments, allies, teacher plants, entheogens,* and *sacred plant medicines,* each carrying a distinct cultural and philosophical weight. I have chosen to use *psychedelic* because it includes both natural and synthetic substances and is widely understood. I use the word *psychedelic* to honor both the modern usage of *psyche* (mind) and its deeper meaning (soul). In English, *soul* may be the closest word we have to mean "spirit embodied on Earth," and this is what I intend to convey through my use of this word. *Delos,* the Greek root of the second part of the word *psychedelic,* means "visible" or "manifest," so I define *psychedelic* as "that which reveals the depth and truth of the soul."

When referring to psychedelic medicines, I am referring to cannabis, psilocybin mushrooms, ayahuasca, and huachuma cactus as well as ketamine, MDMA, and LSD—the medicines most widely available and with which I have the most experience. While I am not including other plant medicines, of which there are many, each with its own richly textured history, or novel psychoactive substances, I believe the majority of what I'm sharing can apply to experiences with those substances as well.

What's possible with psychedelic medicines—what my client Maria experienced, and what countless others are discovering—is rare and precious. An opportunity like this deserves thoughtful preparation, the right setting, trustworthy companions, and adequate time for integration. After reading this book, you will be better prepared to create these conditions for yourself, and in doing so, increase your chances of having a transformative experience.

Healing yourself—bringing compassion to your past, care to your present, and intention to your future—is a journey that requires creativity and great courage. I'm honored to walk this part of the path with you.

CHAPTER 1

How Do Psychedelic Medicines Heal?

"They're gone," he whispered. I was sitting beside a friend an hour after he received his monthly shot of intramuscular ketamine. The voices in his head telling him to end his life had gone away. When he arrived at the clinic, his face had been tight. Now it had softened. The depression he had known since he was a teenager—the nightmarish conglomeration of fatigue, hollowness, and guilt that responded to nothing else—had once again vanished. He would live in peace for another three to four weeks.

Years earlier, in a psychedelic support tent at a festival, I sat beside a woman in her early twenties who had taken a high dose of MDMA. She looked deep into my eyes and spoke with the measured calm of an elder. She put her hand on mine and began telling me the story of her childhood sexual abuse. She had never told this story before. She seemed at peace with the complexity of human nature as she contemplated how sick her abuser must have been. It wasn't forgiveness she was expressing; rather it was a mix of dispassionate honesty, grief, and acceptance. Hearing her composed reflection on such a horrific event astonished me. She was barely out of her teens.

Over the past fifteen years, many people with advanced cancer and long-term AIDS, people staring death in the face and struggling with existential fear and hopelessness, have been given high doses of psilocybin in clinical trials.

After their journeys, most of them said their anxiety had diminished and their fear of death had significantly decreased. Their improved well-being lasted for months.[1]

How are these shifts possible? Do psychedelics create something new in the brain? Do they somehow rewire our memories of painful experiences? Are visions and ego dissolution necessary for transformation? In other words, how in the world do psychedelics catalyze healing?

During my three years teaching psychedelic facilitation through the University of California, Berkeley's certificate program, this question arose regularly. Our instructional team included a medical doctor, two therapists, an interfaith chaplain, a professor of education, a clinically trained medicine woman, and me, all of us seasoned psychedelic facilitators. When we began discussing how psychedelics heal, we discovered we had vastly different perspectives. In fact, many of us had never made our beliefs explicit until our teaching required us to articulate what we'd each taken as self-evident.

If you're considering psychedelics for healing, understanding how they work isn't just intellectual curiosity; it's practical preparation. If you think you can only heal after having a mystical experience, you may be disappointed, as not everyone has one. If you believe healing results purely from altered brain chemistry, it's tempting to approach the experience passively, hoping this novel "treatment" will automatically fix you. When it doesn't work as expected, you could easily become frustrated and wonder, "Why didn't it do the thing?"

Your beliefs about how psychedelics work can shape what you pay attention to during a journey and how you respond when strong emotions surface. For instance, if intense fear arises, you might be tempted to push it away; who wants to feel that? Yet that moment could be a portal to profound healing—if you can recognize it for what it is. Understanding that psychedelics amplify what is already present, and that your attention directs the medicine, can change how you approach the entire experience.

The truth is, there are multiple pathways through which psychedelics can catalyze healing. I think it's valuable to consider several of these pathways so you can set realistic expectations and make the most of your precious opportunity.

You don't need to adopt any single framework. But familiarizing yourself with these perspectives will help you show up prepared for whatever emerges.

I'll begin with the scientific view of the brain as the body's command center and neuroplasticity as one agent of change. Then I'll explain psychedelics' capacity to amplify what's already present in your body and mind. I'll explore the much-discussed mystical experience and how it can shift the way you see yourself and reality. I'll also look at how psychedelics offer healing by deepening your connection with fellow humans and the natural world.

Even if you think you know how psychedelic healing works, I think you'll learn something new. After all, that may be what you're coming for—a new way of looking at the world.

The Scientific View: Your Brain on Psychedelics

Your brain is plastic, or at least it can be. Understanding neuroplasticity is one key to understanding how psychedelics can create change.

Imagine a network of underground tree roots. Over time they grow thick and strong along certain paths, depending on where they found water and nutrients in the past. This root system becomes highly structured, and the roots can't readily change direction once established. Your nervous system has roots too. They are your brain's habitual pathways, also called neural networks. As we age, our brains settle into fixed patterns. While these are efficient adaptations for navigating daily life, they make your brain less flexible than it once was. Depression is a type of patterned thinking in which constant negative thoughts have become fixed pathways that get continually activated.

Psychedelics can be seen as temporarily softening the soil around the roots for days or weeks. The roots don't die or get uprooted, but suddenly they can sense nutrients in new directions. A root that always grew south can suddenly branch east toward water it had never detected before. Roots that have never touched can now find each other and exchange information.

When the soil hardens again, most roots snap back to their old paths. But if a root found something essential in a new direction, like a rich vein of minerals or a water source, that new pathway may stay. The tree will try to reinforce a new pattern if it's useful.

The key lies in what happens while the soil is soft. If you just wait for it to harden again, you will mostly return to the same old root system. But if you consciously send growth toward what you need—toward healing, toward nourishment, toward connection—those new roots have a chance to establish themselves permanently.

How does the soil soften? It starts when the molecules in psychedelic substances fit, like keys, into specific receptors throughout your nervous system, kicking off a cascade of changes, particularly in a network called the default mode network (DMN). If you follow psychedelic clinical trials, you've likely come across this term. The DMN includes regions of the brain tied to who you believe you are and how you think about yourself. It's most active when your attention turns inward, replaying memories, imagining the future, or getting stuck in repetitive thoughts. People who struggle with depression typically show higher activity in this part of the brain.

Brain scans show that classic psychedelics like LSD and psilocybin dramatically lower DMN activity. When the DMN quiets, the rigid thought loops that often plague people with depression and keep us stuck in "the same old me" are interrupted. This decrease in DMN activity frequently accompanies reports of ego dissolution: a temporary loss of the sense of self.

Think of the DMN as the brain's captain. Sometimes the captain becomes overbearing, relentlessly telling you what to do. When you're clinically depressed, it can feel nearly impossible to escape its rule. A classic psychedelic temporarily shuts down this tyrannical commander, allowing the rest of the crew to communicate freely and potentially collaborate in new ways. Parts of the brain that usually work separately—handling sensations, emotions, and memory—begin talking to each other in ways they normally don't. This increase in connection and communication may explain why people report fresh insights and new ways of seeing things during and after psychedelic experiences.

Psychedelics also temporarily change another part of the brain: the amygdala, whose job it is to identify threats. A calmer amygdala lowers your fear response, allowing you to relax and open to the moment. The familiar boundary between self and other softens. An off-duty amygdala also lets you return to painful or traumatic memories with minimal reactivity. However, decreased amygdala activity is why choosing a safe setting and a trustworthy guide is paramount. Your ability to recognize threats and respond effectively will be dampened when your brain is temporarily altered in this way.

These immediate effects of psychedelics—the quieted DMN and the calmer amygdala—don't just change how you feel in the moment. They create a temporary window of neuroplasticity during which your brain becomes unusually open to rewiring.[2] During the few weeks after a psychedelic session, you have a brain that can bend and stretch in new, creative ways. Scientists call this the "critical period," a window of time when your brain is more receptive to novel learning. For people with depression, this window is especially valuable. Alternative neural connections have often become weakened or have been pruned away, and psychedelics appear to help rebuild them, allowing you to interrupt old patterns and strengthen new pathways. The amount of time this window stays open depends on the medicine ingested; with MDMA and psilocybin, the period lasts around two weeks, while with LSD, it can last up to three weeks. Ketamine shows a shorter window of approximately forty-eight hours.[3]

Contrary to the claims that psychedelic substances harm the brain, research shows that, when used safely, they can keep the brain and nervous system healthy and even help the brain heal after injury. New studies are investigating how psilocybin and other psychedelics might help people with traumatic brain injuries.[4]

It's also possible to have too much of a good thing. There is a range of neuroplasticity that supports brain health and flexibility. However, at a certain point, the brain can become too plastic and chaotic, as seen in some mental illnesses. Psychedelic research is looking to determine where the line between helpful and harmful lies.

Neuroscience helps explain what happens in your brain during a psychedelic experience, but it doesn't fully capture what you might be feeling or how healing unfolds. For that, we need a different lens—one that focuses less on molecules and neural networks and more on what's happening at the level of consciousness.

Consciousness as the Healer: The Amplification Effect

Stanislav Grof, a Czech psychiatrist who conducted thousands of LSD therapy sessions between the 1950s and the 1970s, famously said, "Psychedelics are to the study of the mind what the microscope is to biology and the telescope is to astronomy."[5] This may be part of what makes psychedelic medicines so interesting to therapists and psychologists: They amplify what's present but is hard to see, bringing into sharp focus what is normally hidden or blurry.

Under the influence of psychedelics, it often feels as though your senses open wider, allowing more information in than usual. The sound of a plucked guitar string, the texture of clouds in the sky, or the figures emerging from an abstract painting can become startlingly vivid. You can see dimensions and layers of detail that you never noticed before. A magnificently rich sensory world reveals itself to you.

But psychedelics don't just amplify what's outside you; they also amplify what's inside. Closing your eyes allows you to turn this mechanism inward, directing this amplification toward memories, thoughts, and emotions. While our bodies and minds can make sense of a tremendous amount of information, we have limits. We can't be aware of all of it, all the time. The human brain and psyche, in their effort to help us navigate daily life, are adept at preventing intense feelings from overtaking us. Most of us use some portion of our nervous system's processing power to manage emotions that are right below the surface. These feelings of fear, resentment, or despair can be hazy and elusive.

As a psychedelic medicine relaxes your defenses, you may feel buried emotions or memories beginning to surface and flow, as if a dam has been removed. It's common to feel your inner world more fully, with heightened sensitivity to your emotions and felt sensations. Or you may feel the tension in your body—where you hold it and what beliefs it's connected to—in much finer detail. Previously unnoticed sensations, thoughts, and emotions gets turned up to maximum volume until they fill your perception completely.

During a psychedelic journey, this amplification effect can magnify rage, grief, or insecurity until you feel physically sick and need to purge, whether by vocalizing, heading to the bathroom, or even vomiting. This release can also be subtle, with tears or shivering, like tension slowly unwinding. Some healing traditions have long recognized and reframed this potentially uncomfortable purging as "getting well," a welcome purification.

While it can be excruciating to come into contact with the tangled layers of emotional wounds, if you stay with them, something surprising can happen. By directing your attention to the pain and staying present, it can shift or even relax, as though it has simply been waiting to be acknowledged. It's as though your attention, your awareness itself, is part of the medicine.

I once worked with a young woman, Alexis, who had been through a few rounds of chemotherapy for stomach cancer. When she was finally stable and in remission, she wanted to experience a mushroom journey to look at her fear of death, since she knew it was taking a toll on her. She told me that her fear felt like a virus, constantly present and affecting her ability to enjoy her life. During her journey, she began growling and pounding the ground beside her. Her voice got louder and louder, and she clenched her fists. Finally, a scream came out, and she began to cry.

During her first integration session, she explained that on her journey, she had seen her fear represented as a dial. She watched as it rose from 40 percent to 100 percent, until it became so intense she had to scream. She realized that her resistance to fully feeling it was actually making it worse. After her journey, she reported feeling immense spaciousness. Although the fear wasn't completely gone, it felt workable. It wasn't in charge anymore.

INNER HEALING INTELLIGENCE

If awareness is part of the medicine, then what directs your attention to a specific memory, emotion, or tension? Many psychedelic therapists believe in a natural impulse toward healing. According to this idea, it's not primarily the molecules and brain changes that catalyze healing; instead, healing emerges when you create the inner and outer conditions that support your body and consciousness to heal themselves. This perspective suggests that resolving emotional wounds and processing trauma at the level of consciousness may result in a reorganized brain and body, rather than the other way around.

This concept isn't new. The understanding that natural forces within us are the true healers, known in Latin as *vis medicatrix naturae* (the healing power of nature), is ancient wisdom that informs many schools of traditional and alternative healing.[6]

Stanislav Grof coined the term *inner healing intelligence* after years of observing this phenomenon during psychedelic sessions. Just as a fractured bone will mend itself when correctly set, a fractured psyche or heart, when given the right conditions, will do its best to heal. Psychedelics create these conditions by temporarily loosening our psychological defenses and helping our bodies relax. Our psyche somehow knows how to bring the most pressing wounds or neglected parts of ourselves to the surface first. This is not an intellectual decision; it's the manifestation of a deeper drive toward healthy reorganization and ongoing integration.

In a safe, supportive setting, people can spontaneously begin to relive painful or incomplete experiences from their past. In this psychedelic catharsis, people don't just recall intense emotions and physical sensations mentally; they often reexperience them in the body. The difference is that they can now process those experiences with adult awareness, allowing previously bound-up energy to be released and finally digested. Trusting this spontaneous healing force informs the nondirective facilitation approach to psychedelic healing, which I explain in greater detail in chapter 4.

Healing Through Connection

Healing rarely happens in isolation. It often deepens when witnessed and held by others. Many of us carry some degree of relational wounding or trauma. Early painful experiences imprint on young developing brains. We respond to these experiences, and they often continue to shape how we approach relationships throughout our lives. If the original wounding happened in a relationship, the healing of the wound usually needs to happen through relationship as well.

This relational healing can show up in different ways. Many people find that during and after their experiences with psychedelics, they make deeper contact with themselves—their bodies, emotions, memories, dreams, and visions. Connection with friends, family, and even strangers may feel easier. You can enjoy a greater sense of closeness with the person sitting with you, which is one reason having a trained guide by your side can be so valuable. Even if your companion speaks no words but keeps you protected while exuding warmth and care, their presence alone can be healing. If your guide is also a trained therapist or skilled in psychological healing, the healing potential is even greater.

This capacity for connection extends beyond your human relationships. During a psychedelic journey, you may experience intimacy with an oak tree, a hummingbird, a fox, the sunlight, the smell of rain, the twinkling stars, or the rising crescent moon. Many people find their eyes and hearts open to the world in a way they remember from childhood. It is as though we can sense the aliveness radiating from within all of creation and feel drawn into more intimate contact with the world. When psychedelic medicines spark this recognition of belonging to the sacred web of life, mechanical, scientific explanations of life in which each species fits into its own isolated box no longer suffice. Treating fellow beings and the living world as resources to be exploited becomes painful. Reconnection with a sacred world, which often feels more like a remembering than a revelation, is a healing salve for any soul aching from disconnection.

The Mystical Experience

Relational healing can extend beyond human and planetary connection. For some people, psychedelics open a door to something even more vast: an encounter with the sacred itself.

In a follow-up study at New York University, a cancer patient who had a high-dose psilocybin journey reflected on her experience by saying, "There was something on top of the mountain. Call it God, call it some divine entity. . . . It was like a spiritual calling." Another reflected: "I was the cloud, I was everything, and that was the theme throughout . . . that I was all this, this was me. And it was so wonderful."[7]

In a later study, Johns Hopkins University and New York University invited twenty-nine clergy members from Christian, Jewish, Islamic, and Buddhist traditions to take psilocybin under careful scientific supervision. After weeks of preparation, each participant received two moderate- to high-dose sessions. The results were striking: 88 percent of participants reported a "complete mystical experience" during at least one of their sessions. While half of them described their experience as "psychologically challenging," nearly all said their psilocybin journey ranked among the five most spiritually significant experiences of their lives.[8]

Six months later, participants reported sustained changes in their lives: deeper experiences of prayer, greater effectiveness as spiritual leaders, and newfound appreciation for other faith traditions. Their sense of the sacred in daily life intensified, and their religious vocations felt renewed. A year later, the changes persisted.

The mystical experience is defined as a sense of connection with something larger than our everyday selves. This includes a reconnection with the natural and more-than-human worlds, but also extends to experiences that can only be described as transcendent. Mystical experiences during psychedelic journeys can be truly numinous, shifting your view of reality in an instant. There's a reason people often call them "ineffable"—they feel impossible to put into words. If you've prayed to God your entire life, a full-blown visionary encounter with the divine can be life-changing. If you haven't, even more so.

Clinical studies show that mystical experiences tend to occur at doses of about 20–30 milligrams of pure psilocybin (approximately 2–5 grams of dried mushrooms, depending on potency).[9] Some historians and authors have surmised that ecstatic experiences initiated by psychedelics or other practices are the source of ancient religious visions and prophecies. They believe these experiences may exist at the root of early spiritual traditions that grew into organized religions.[10] Whether or not psychedelics sparked ancient revelations, the healing potential of mystical experiences is undeniable.

What initiates a mystical experience during a psychedelic journey? Ultimately, it remains a mystery. After such an experience, most people lose interest in understanding *why* it happened. It's like falling in love: You don't wonder why or how it happened. You're too busy being in love.

RECONCILING OUR FEAR OF DEATH

One of the most striking effects of a mystical experience is its capacity to transform our relationship with death. How much of our pain and insecurity is rooted in the reality of impermanence? Nobody wants to talk about death, but it might be the one thing we all have in common. The thought of it brings up so much: regrets; fear of being apart from the people we love; and fear of the unknown or of losing control. It's the ultimate loss: letting go of both body and life.

A high-dose psilocybin journey can be intensely challenging. A temporary death of the ego and dissolution of everything you thought you were is no easy ride. If psychedelic experiences can help us practice letting go so completely, might they prepare us for the ultimate letting go? If we can learn to surrender to the dissolution of self during a journey, we may find ourselves less afraid when death itself arrives. This is one reason why I believe access to supported psychedelic experiences for people facing terminal diagnoses should be prioritized.

Studies show the value of even one session. Tom, a fifty-year-old man with chronic myeloid leukemia and chronic anxiety, described a sense of all-knowingness during his psilocybin journey, saying, "There is nothing to fear after you stop being in your body. . . . It's absolutely no hell or heaven. It's just nothing to be afraid of." He described being surrounded by an "overwhelming feeling of love." In a follow-up interview, he said: "I don't have a fear of death. . . . I am more interested in life now than ever before. . . . Death in itself does not scare me."[11]

After these experiences, many participants report their anxiety either decreased or vanished completely. They also report being more open to continuity after death and to the possibility that some kind of all-loving presence awaits us. What could be more healing than that?

Ancestral Inheritance

Research into transgenerational trauma has shown that intense experiences endured by one generation can produce symptoms in their descendants.[12] As survivors of the transatlantic slave trade, the Armenian genocide, the Holocaust, and other historical traumas confirm, the memories of those horrors live within the descendants of the survivors in ways that are hard to measure but impossible to ignore. I have worked with clients whose symptoms make no sense if you look at their individual biography but make much more sense when they share the life stories of their parents and grandparents.

During psychedelic journeys, some people encounter what feels like ancestral material, including grief, rage, and visionary imagery that doesn't seem to belong to their own life history. Whether these experiences represent actual contact with inherited memory or are the psyche's way of making sense of patterns passed down through family systems, many people find they shift how they understand their history, and this increases their compassion. This is worth exploring in integration. When you consider your own health, you might ask: "How healthy were my parents or grandparents physically, psychologically, and emotionally? What suffering did they endure? How might their experiences still be affecting me?"

Beyond Medication: Wider Circles of Healing

All of these mechanisms—from neuroplasticity to amplification to mystical experience to transgenerational healing—point to a simple truth: Psychedelics work differently from conventional medications.

While psychedelic healing can *sometimes* be a direct result of the substance itself, more often these medicines work by helping you engage with memories and intense emotions in your body and mind. The symptom reduction is an effect of the work you do during the medicine session and in the weeks that follow. Psychedelics can help you identify areas of your life that require attention, release stagnant emotions, and come into a more honest relationship with others and with yourself. While they occasionally provide immediate symptom relief, this is rare. Instead, you're more likely to gain insight into the underlying causes driving your symptoms and be offered creative new perspectives on your habitual thoughts, your interactions with the people you love, and the impacts of the semiconscious choices you make throughout the day. In this way, psychedelics work more like therapy, massage, or acupuncture. You use them for a period of time to shift habitual patterns in your body or mind, often needing them less and less frequently over time.

Using psychedelic medicines for healing isn't new. Indigenous communities across the world have been working with psychoactive plant medicines for thousands of years as part of their healing and spiritual practices. These medicines, which include psilocybin mushrooms, ayahuasca, sacred cacti, and cannabis, are never seen as stand-alone treatments but rather as sacraments woven into larger ceremonial contexts. In ritual settings, trained healers guide people through experiences to address physical illnesses, emotional wounds, spiritual disconnection, and community conflicts. The healing typically isn't limited to the individual; ceremonies often strengthen bonds within the community and reinforce individuals' connections to the land and their ancestors.

Modern science is only now catching up to these traditions, with major universities launching psychedelic research programs in recent years. If you follow psychedelic science news, you've likely seen numerous studies suggesting impressive results. As of this book's publication, universities around the world are recruiting participants for dozens of clinical trials studying psilocybin, MDMA, LSD, and ketamine for conditions including obsessive-compulsive disorder, chronic pain, PTSD, depression, and end-of-life anxiety.[13]

In my experience, it's not a single psychedelic journey or even a series of journeys that bring about lasting change. Psychedelics are not a magic cure or a ticket to sudden enlightenment. They will not instantaneously save you or deliver you from your suffering. On the contrary, they are likely to show you both the blessings and the burdens of your life—in Technicolor.

You now have multiple ways to consider how psychedelics catalyze healing: changes in the brain, amplification of what's present, innate healing intelligence, relational connection, mystical experience, reconciliation with death, and healing across generations. These aren't separate mechanisms but interwoven possibilities that may all be part of your journey. The rest of this book is dedicated to helping you access this potential as fully as possible and with minimal risk. Healing doesn't happen to you; it happens through you.

CHAPTER 2

Psychedelic Safety: What You Need to Know

Humans have been using psychedelic medicines for thousands of years. They're woven into the fabric of our shared history, helping us seek connection and meaning. And yet, while these medicines offer real potential for healing and exploration, they're not without risk.

Risk is different from harm: It's the possibility that something might go wrong. Some risks are greater than others, and some affect certain people more than others. We accept risk in nearly every part of life. We drive on busy freeways; we undergo medical procedures; we eat food prepared by people we don't know. Understanding what might go wrong doesn't mean you need to live in fear. It means you can make better choices about what you're getting into and prepare yourself.

In the following pages, I'll give you accurate information, up-to-date and vetted, on what you need to know about medical conditions, mental health, and the actual physical risks of taking psychedelic substances into your body. For most people, psychological risks matter more than physical risks and are worth understanding. I'll offer a reframe for "bad trips" and share what I believe is essential for those who have experienced trauma to know. I'll also describe the changing legal landscape: which countries and US states have decriminalized or legalized psychedelics and what that means for you.

Medical Screening Comes First

The primary physical risk with psychedelic substances comes from how they interact with particular health issues or medications. If you have any serious medical concerns, consult with a medical professional first. The conditions that require the greatest care are heart problems, including high blood pressure or previous heart attacks; seizures; kidney or liver issues; and substance use disorders. Many prescription medications and supplements also have serious interactions with psychedelic substances. To help determine if you may have a contraindicated condition, take my "Psychedelic Readiness Self-Assessment" in appendix A.

Screening is the first step in determining whether psychedelics are right for you right now. A thorough screening should cover your medical history, current medications, mental health diagnoses, family mental health history, social history, and current life circumstances. If you are working with a facilitator and they don't ask you these questions up front, it's a red flag. If you choose to take psychedelics on your own or with a sitter, you need to think this through yourself or seek a medical consultation. Be honest. Hiding information to get access can put you at real risk, so find a trustworthy psychedelic guide or a psychedelic-knowledgeable medical provider you feel safe with.

MENTAL HEALTH HISTORY AND RISK

Psychedelics can trigger or worsen mental illness. That said, do psychedelics cause schizophrenia? The research says no.[1] People with no family history rarely develop schizophrenia after a psychedelic experience. However, for people who already carry a genetic risk or have other risk factors for schizophrenia, symptoms can be triggered by psychedelics or other powerful experiences that dramatically alter consciousness. These individuals should not use these substances.

Other conditions that rule out or seriously limit what may be safe to explore include schizoaffective or bipolar I disorder, active suicidal thoughts, or a history of psychosis during depression: seeing or hearing things that aren't there or having beliefs disconnected from reality.

If you or a close family member has experienced manic episodes (periods of elevated mood, racing thoughts, risky behavior, or reduced need for sleep), psychedelics aren't necessarily ruled out, but you need a thorough medical evaluation first. You should be stable for at least three years before considering taking psychedelics other than ketamine in a supervised setting, and you need a professional assessment from a psychiatrist familiar with psychedelics to be cleared to do so. Even if you are cleared to proceed, always start with a low dose in a safe setting with experienced support.

Physical Risks

Can taking a psychedelic substance kill you? It's highly unlikely. Scientists measure toxicity using what's called an LD_{50}, or median lethal dose, which is the amount of a substance needed to kill half of a test group of animals. This statistic lets us compare the toxicity of different substances.

Deaths from psilocybin mushrooms are vanishingly rare.[2] The LD_{50} is 280 milligrams per kilogram of body weight (mg/kg). For a 150-pound person, that's 19,000 mg of pure psilocybin. But most people eat dried mushrooms, not the isolated compound. Though potency varies, the average is 7 mg per dried gram, meaning you'd need to eat over five pounds of dried mushrooms—five hundred times the typical dose for a strong experience—to approach the lethal amount.

As for LSD, no fatalities have been recorded as a direct result of ingesting the substance alone, even though there are documented cases of people accidentally taking a thousand or more times a normal dose. Based on animal experiments, the estimated LD_{50} for LSD in humans is around 50 mg, five hundred times the normal therapeutic dose of 100 *micro*grams. As one study notes, "Even taking this theoretical value for granted, it is difficult to think of drugs or medicines that, when administered 100 or 200 times their therapeutic dose, do not cause serious damage to the health of the individual."[3]

THE DANGERS OF CONTAMINATION

That said, these numbers only apply to pure substances. One of the most serious physical risks today is contamination. Synthetic psychedelics like ketamine, MDMA, and other powdered substances not obtained through a pharmacy could be contaminated with fentanyl or other unknown adulterants. Fentanyl is deadly in tiny amounts, and it sometimes shows up in white powder substances. While contamination is rare, it can kill you.

If you are planning to use any powdered substances or trusting anyone else to serve one, test for fentanyl first. You can buy fentanyl test strips online or through harm reduction organizations. They're inexpensive and simple to use. Because fentanyl can clump together, one dose might test negative even when some is present elsewhere in the same bag. Make sure to crush and thoroughly mix the entire batch before dissolving a portion to test. Even so, it is safest to test every portion. Additional precautions:

- Never use a new substance alone.
- Always start with a small amount to test potency.
- Have Narcan (naloxone) available anywhere white powders are being used in case of overdose from fentanyl contamination. You can purchase it online.
- Know that most US states have Good Samaritan laws, which legally protect people who seek medical help for someone experiencing an overdose from being arrested.

DESIGNER DRUGS: EXPERIMENTING ON YOURSELF

Another concern is designer drugs. As synthetic psychedelics are banned, new ones are promptly created to circumvent prohibition, creating a cycle that makes substances less safe, not more. These substances are called designer drugs or research chemicals and can be purchased online. When people buy these, they are trusting a lab they don't know in an unknown country to send them what's advertised. But because these are brand-new compounds, there's no way to test the purity or potency of these substances. They can be sold as another substance that looks identical while having a completely different molecular identity and effects. Experienced users can usually tell the difference, but newer users can't. Sometimes nothing bad happens, and other times people die. If you order unknown powders online, you're experimenting on yourself.

MDMA'S UNIQUE DANGERS

MDMA carries physical risks that other psychedelics don't. In hot, crowded environments such as clubs and festivals where you are dancing for hours, it can interfere with your body's ability to regulate temperature, which can rise to dangerous levels. Consuming alcohol or other drugs, including cocaine, amphetamines, or cathinones, can further elevate your temperature, increasing the chance of unpredictable and toxic effects.

Hyperthermia—dangerously high body temperature—can cause organ failure and death. Early warning signs include confusion, severe headache, nausea, rapid heartbeat, and feeling extremely hot. If someone shows these symptoms, get them to a cool place, provide water, and seek medical help immediately.

Drinking too much water is another danger. MDMA makes you thirsty, but drinking excessive water can cause hyponatremia or water intoxication, which can also be fatal. The guideline is roughly one pint (500 ml) of water per hour, which is plenty to stay hydrated.

These risks drop significantly when MDMA is taken in controlled settings at therapeutic doses.

THE RISKS OF MIXING MEDICINES

Some people like to mix psychedelic substances, called layering or stacking. Someone might pair LSD with mushrooms, ketamine with cannabis, or MDMA with huachuma cactus, reporting that the combination creates an enhanced experience with more depth. But mixing some substances introduces new risks.

Every batch of every substance varies in strength unless it's been made in a pharmacy or tested in a lab. When you combine substances, you create unpredictable effects. The safe approach is to use a single substance multiple times before considering mixing it with anything else. It's good to know the potency and felt effects of every new batch of any substance, synthetic or natural, before combining it with anything else. Some combinations can kill you:[4]

- **Depressants** such as ketamine, alcohol, opioids, and benzodiazepines are substances that slow your nervous system. They all slow your breathing and heart rate. Mix them and you can stop breathing. This is how most overdose deaths happen: not from one substance, but from combining depressants. Most are unintentional.
- **Stimulants** are substances that speed up your system, like MDMA, methamphetamine, or even high doses of caffeine. They put extreme stress on your heart. When combined, you risk panic attacks, dangerously high heart rate and blood pressure, overheating, stroke, or heart attack.
- **MAOIs** (monoamine oxidase inhibitors), found in ayahuasca, block certain enzymes in your body. When combined with stimulants, many common medications, or substances that affect serotonin, they can be fatal.
- **MDMA and other substances that affect serotonin** are also dangerous to combine with certain antidepressants, which in extreme cases can cause serotonin syndrome, a potentially deadly condition where too much serotonin builds up in your body.

Never combine substances without testing their potency and researching their interactions. When in doubt, don't mix. Be equally cautious when someone offers you a combination—always ask what's in it and research the combination yourself before taking it. Organizations like TripSit and PsychonautWiki provide detailed information about drug interactions and safe use.[5]

WHEN VISUALS DON'T GO AWAY

In rare cases, visual disturbances from a psychedelic experience don't fully go away. This condition, called hallucinogen persisting perception disorder (HPPD), involves persistent perceptual changes like visual snow, trails, halos, geometric patterns, or afterimages. It's a neurological issue related to changes in how your brain processes visual information.

HPPD is more common with frequent use, higher doses, and mixing substances (especially cannabis), and it appears more often with LSD than psilocybin. For most people it fades over months to a couple of years. For some it becomes permanent. While uncommon, it's worth knowing this can happen, especially if you're considering repeated or high-dose experiences.

THE RISK OF ACCIDENTS

Assuming you have medical clearance and your medicine is clean, appropriately dosed for potency, and taken by itself, the physical risks are minimal. But your environment is another matter. Most injuries and deaths related to psychedelics result from falling, drowning, or car accidents.[6] Altered states of consciousness can distort your awareness of your surroundings and affect your judgment, leading to risky behavior, especially without supervision. As mentioned, because psychedelics temporarily change the part of your brain that normally assesses threats, they can dramatically lower your sense of fear. This lowered vigilance can help you access and heal traumatic memories and encourages bonding, yet without someone sober keeping watch, it's possible to unknowingly make dangerous decisions.

You can avoid this risk by preparing your environment carefully and having a sober person—ideally someone trained or experienced—with you throughout your journey. I'll compare settings in the next chapter, but the short version is: Living rooms are good, and the woods can be okay if it's a familiar spot. The ocean or other bodies of water are not advised, and alone in a hot tub is a bad idea.

Don't drive for twenty-four hours after an experience, and only after you've had a full night of rest. Visual distortions and impaired judgment can last for hours afterward. Have someone sober drive if you need to go anywhere.

Psychological Risks

While the physical risk of psychedelics is low after proper screening, psychological risks are a bigger and more complex concern. Psychedelics can cut through layers of psychological defenses and open you to hidden parts of yourself. This openness creates both healing potential and vulnerability.

DIFFICULT EXPERIENCES VERSUS BAD TRIPS

The term *bad trip* has been around for decades, and people have stories of seriously nightmarish experiences. Even years later, they'll exclaim, "Never again!" But if you ask what happened, the story often includes a dose that was too high for their level of preparation and inadequate support.

Bad trips often happen when someone is younger or more psychologically fragile. Being thrust into an intense and disorienting state of consciousness with no familiar reference points can evoke terror that the experience will never end, or that you will go crazy or die. This fear can be intensified in unprepared settings such as at school, a friend's house, or a party. Or the setting may be safe, but because the dose is higher than appropriate, its effects become overwhelming and terrifying.

When someone has a frightening psychedelic experience in an intentional setting with good support, they are more likely to describe it as a "difficult experience" rather than a bad trip. Wrestling with shame, grief, rage, or terror for five hours—and being unable to get out of it—is a hard way to spend a day. But psychedelics themselves don't create these emotions. As mentioned, psychedelics often amplify what's already present in your body and mind. That might sound agonizing, but when emotions are amplified, they also become more accessible and possible to work with, especially with good support. For many people, what surfaces during these intense moments is unprocessed trauma. In chapter 7, I offer suggestions for navigating fear and other strong emotions during a psychedelic experience.

WHEN YOUR DEFENSES ARE DOWN

Psychedelics can make you highly suggestible. Your usual filters and critical thinking can become dramatically reduced or dissolve entirely. At the same time, your brain's ability to find patterns and create meaning goes into overdrive. This isn't just a side effect: When the inputs you absorb are intentional, positive, and directed toward health, suggestibility can be integral to these medicines' therapeutic potential.

But the same openness that allows you to let go of rigid beliefs and access healing also makes you vulnerable to outside influences. You can't get one without the other. This is why your choice of setting and companions is critical—a topic I return to throughout this book.

PSYCHEDELICS AND TRAUMA

What we call "trauma" refers to what happens in the body after surviving an event that exceeds what your nervous system could handle in the moment. This can be a specific event, such as a fire, a car accident, or a violent encounter. But trauma can also result from the chronic stress of growing up in a neglectful or abusive home or from fearing for your safety because of your gender, race, religion, or sexual orientation. Fighting to exist or collapsing under the pressure of relentless vigilance is exhausting and takes a massive toll on the body. Your body survives by compartmentalizing what it can't process in the moment. In their 2022 book *The Myth of Normal,* authors Gabor Maté and Daniel Maté define trauma as "a psychic injury, lodged in our nervous system, mind, and body, lasting long past the original incident(s), triggerable at any moment. It is a constellation of hardships, composed of the wound itself and the residual burdens that our woundedness imposes on our bodies and souls."[7]

A common survival response to trauma is disconnection, often called dissociation. This occurs when your nervous system blocks out everything not immediately necessary for survival. When you repeatedly dissociate, it can become automatic, potentially changing how your brain works. Long-term effects of trauma include anxiety, depression, and physical health problems as well as disconnection from yourself and others.

The degree to which a traumatic event affects you is subjective, regardless of how "bad" the event may appear to others. For example, being bitten by a small aggressive dog might be easy for an adult to process, but it could be terrifying for a young child, leading to a lifelong fear of dogs. But beyond individual differences, recent trauma research shows that what determines whether an event becomes traumatic isn't primarily the intensity of the experience itself but rather how well you were supported by your loved ones or community in its immediate aftermath.

CAN PSYCHEDELICS HEAL TRAUMA?

Much of the research on psychedelics has focused on their potential to help resolve symptoms of PTSD. Some people avoid psychedelic medicines because they are rightly concerned that the experience will trigger or aggravate their trauma symptoms. Other people with trauma histories dive into medicine journeys with abandon, hoping for relief from their symptoms. So when are psychedelics helpful for someone with trauma, and when are they potentially harmful?

This is a complex question. Expanded states are intimately related to trauma. In fact, a traumatic experience that causes extreme fear or dissociation could be considered a type of expanded state. Taking a psychedelic and having your consciousness expand can "remind" your nervous system of past dissociation and bring a traumatic memory back to the surface. This is part of psychedelics' trauma healing potential. If the experience takes place in a safe setting with a skilled guide or companion, the memory can be worked with effectively. Otherwise, unleashing traumatic memories without proper support can be destabilizing and even retraumatizing.

WHICH MEDICINE FOR WHICH TRAUMA?

We could safely say that some psychedelic medicines help some people with some kinds of trauma. Ketamine and MDMA tend to be gentler starting points. Ketamine creates distance from painful material, letting you examine it with less emotional charge, while MDMA quiets the fear response. Classic psychedelics like psilocybin, LSD, and ayahuasca are different. While they can sometimes dramatically shift your relationship to traumatic memories, they are unpredictable. Symptoms may flare before settling, and some people find themselves worse off afterward. I discuss each medicine's relationship to trauma in more detail in chapter 5.

If you have trauma in your personal or family history, consider starting with ketamine or MDMA. If you want to work with a more powerful psychedelic, get an individual assessment and find a trauma-trained facilitator who will give you their full attention, include thorough preparation and integration, and start you at a low dose. Do not journey alone. If something opens up but isn't well supported or completed, you may end up worse off than before.

Are Psychedelics Addictive?

Given the decades of antidrug propaganda we've been exposed to, it's understandable that people worry about addiction, also known as substance use disorder. You might wonder whether psychedelic substances are addictive themselves or whether using them could trigger a relapse if there is a history of substance abuse. These concerns make sense, especially if you or someone you love has struggled with addiction.

Many contemporary addiction researchers are pushing back against the conventional narrative that says taking psychoactive substances permanently changes your brain or causes dependency.[8] The *Diagnostic and Statistical Manual of Mental Disorders*, 5th edition (DSM-5) defines hallucinogen use disorder, similar to other substance disorders, as compulsive use that results in unsuccessful attempts to cut down usage, neglected responsibilities, relationship problems, isolation, putting yourself in danger, and using despite harm to your physical and mental health.[9] Addiction is defined by compulsion causing harm, not only by frequency of use. Even if you regularly use a substance, if you're functional, keeping up with your responsibilities, maintaining relationships, and taking care of your body, it may not be a problem. For a full list of symptoms defining substance use disorder, see "Substance Use" in appendix A.

WHY CLASSIC PSYCHEDELICS AREN'T ADDICTIVE

LSD and psilocybin have close to zero risk of addiction. Your body builds tolerance so quickly that repeated use becomes unrewarding.[10] On top of that, after a high-dose experience, people rarely want another one soon. In fact, a common refrain after a journey is "That was amazing, but I'm never doing it again." As the benefits unfold over the coming days and weeks, the sentiment often changes to, "Well, maybe I'll do it again. But not for a while." Most people need time to integrate their experience. It's intense and far from an escape. As a result, physical addiction to LSD or psilocybin is essentially unheard of, and psychological addiction is almost as rare. I have seen a few people over the years use them in a way that seemed compulsive and like an attempt to avoid reality. But this is the exception.

People in many traditional cultures have maintained ongoing relationships with ayahuasca, peyote, and psilocybin mushrooms for thousands of years. Again, the question isn't whether you use these medicines regularly, but whether that use is causing harm in your life. If the answer is no—if your relationships are strong, your physical health is stable, and you're fulfilling your commitments and maintaining an active and creative life while staying involved in your community—then regular use may not be a problem.

HIGHER-RISK SUBSTANCES: MDMA, KETAMINE, AND CANNABIS

MDMA, ketamine, and cannabis, however, do carry some risk of compulsive use. Ketamine numbs pain, and people can end up using it compulsively. MDMA is considered an entactogen or an empathogen, but is related to amphetamine and has stimulant effects that some people can become dependent on. Cannabis can become addictive as well. If you have a history of addiction, use these substances only in supervised settings with professional support. The same applies if you're in recovery. Though rare, these substances can trigger relapse, so it's best to work with a practitioner who understands both psychedelics and addiction.

For people without an addiction history, these substances still require careful attention to frequency. Many people use ketamine every three or four weeks as an effective antidepressant. They depend on it, but their quality of life is significantly improved. Dependency isn't automatically a problem if it's not causing harm. The idea that we shouldn't depend on substances is unrealistic.

The Legal Landscape

Laws prohibiting psychedelic substances remain in place throughout much of the world, with possession punishable by fines, felony charges, and prison time, and, in some countries, by death. If you don't want to be fined or jailed, learn your local laws, and make sure you understand the difference between decriminalization and legalization. Consider your risks carefully, understand the legal consequences of your choices, and decide how you want to proceed.

Since the early 2000s, the legal status of psychedelic medicines has shifted dramatically in the United States and around the world. Many countries are choosing saner approaches. Some countries have decriminalized possession and personal use, while others have moved toward legal, regulated access.[11]

LEGAL AND PROTECTED USE

Several countries protect the traditional and religious use of plant medicines. Peru, Bolivia, and Brazil legally protect ayahuasca, used by Indigenous and mestizo people for traditional healing ceremonies throughout the Amazon rainforest and by religious groups that revere it as their sacrament. Countries throughout Africa actively protect or don't regulate the *iboga* plant and ibogaine, which have been used in Indigenous ceremonies for generations. In Mexico, the ceremonial use of psilocybin mushrooms and 5-MeO-DMT is protected by law, while ibogaine remains unregulated. In the United States, the peyote cactus has been protected for Native American religious use since the 1970s, and each year, more plant-medicine churches receive federal exemptions allowing them to legally use ayahuasca in ceremonies. Some countries have never prohibited psilocybin mushrooms. They are legal to possess and use in Jamaica, the Bahamas, and the British Virgin Islands.

Medical pathways are opening as well. Australia now allows MDMA to be prescribed for PTSD and psilocybin for depression when the patient hasn't responded to other treatments.[12] Canada allows health care practitioners to request psilocybin mushrooms and MDMA for patients with serious or life-threatening conditions.[13] Ketamine clinics offering treatment for anxiety, depression, and chronic pain have opened across the United States, Canada, Europe, Africa, and East Asia.

DECRIMINALIZATION AND STATE-LEVEL LEGALIZATION

Decriminalization means that possession of a substance is not a criminal offense, although the substance remains technically illegal. Portugal has led the way by decriminalizing possession of all drugs in 2001. Switzerland and Spain have also implemented drug policy reform and relaxed their laws. In all three countries there has been no notable increase in usage.[14] The Czech Republic has decriminalized possession of psilocybin mushrooms, LSD, and other psychedelics, while Canada's British Columbia province has decriminalized personal use of MDMA. The Netherlands has legalized psilocybin-containing truffles.

In the United States, change is happening state by state and city by city. Oregon, Colorado, and New Mexico have legalized psilocybin mushrooms, with regulations unfolding in real time. However, even though substances are legal on the state level, they are still illegal at the federal level, and the FBI and DEA still treat possession as a criminal offense.

Mushrooms and certain psychedelic plant medicines have been decriminalized in cities including Washington, D.C., Denver, Oakland, and Seattle.[15] Similarly, even though substances may be decriminalized in a city, they may still be illegal at the state level, meaning that state-level law enforcement, like the highway patrol, still treats possession as a criminal offense.

HOW LEGALIZATION IMPROVES SAFETY

When substances are regulated, testing becomes standard, as it has for psilocybin in Oregon and Colorado. Test results confirm purity and potency, reducing the risk of contamination or taking a stronger dose than intended. This precision decreases the likelihood of overdose. Most people aren't looking to get obliterated. They just want the right amount.

Another immediate benefit of legalization is decreasing the harm of policing and incarcerating people for the substances they choose to put into their bodies. These laws disproportionately hurt people of color, unhoused populations, and people with less money, as they face a higher risk of illegal searches and seizures. This results in higher incarceration rates and long-term consequences for already marginalized people.

With regulation, safer spaces become available for people to access these medicines, such as the licensed service centers that have opened in Oregon for facilitated psilocybin sessions. Regulation also removes the stigma that causes people to hide a part of their life that matters deeply to them. Many highly functional, engaged contributors to society conceal their psychedelic use for fear of being shunned or losing their jobs, even though psychedelics have only improved their lives. Compelling arguments abound for psychedelics—and all drugs, for that matter—to be fully legalized and regulated, or at the very least, decriminalized.

Reducing Your Risk

The following recommendations apply whether you're planning to work with a guide, attend a ceremony, or explore on your own.

- If you have any physical or mental health conditions or take any medications, talk to a medical doctor knowledgeable about psychedelics first.
- Only use psychedelics when you're physically healthy and emotionally stable.
- Make sure your substances are pure and start by taking one at a time. If layering, only use combinations that have been proven safe.
- Don't take psychedelics alone until you have extensive experience. Have someone sober with you.

- Prepare for your experience.
- Use them in a familiar, safe environment.
- Dosage: Start low and go slow. You can always take more, but you can't take less.
- Don't watch the news or violent movies, listen to disturbing music, or expose yourself to anything you wouldn't show to a child. This applies right before, during, and after your experience.
- Eat, drink, and rest afterward.
- Don't drive or operate machinery for at least twenty-four hours and only after a full night of sleep.
- Give yourself time to integrate your experience.

IN CASE OF AN EMERGENCY

For true medical emergencies during a psychedelic experience—such as difficulty breathing, chest pain, or loss of consciousness—always seek immediate medical attention. This might mean calling 911, going directly to an emergency room, or having a trusted person drive you to urgent care, depending on your circumstances and what feels safest for you and your community.

Always tell emergency responders what substance was taken and how much. In most US states, if you take someone to the hospital or call 911, regardless of the substance they have taken and how you are involved, Good Samaritan laws protect you from arrest.

Navigating Risk Wisely

The physical, psychological, and legal risks of psychedelics are real and need to be thoughtfully considered. If your life is already chaotic or unstable, it may not be the right time for a journey. And despite what some psychedelic enthusiasts might say, not everyone should take them. Some nervous systems are too fragile, and some lives lack the stability and support needed to process what these medicines can surface. To evaluate your personal readiness for psychedelics and review a list of alternatives, see appendix A.

Even if you are fit to proceed, my suggestion is to gradually build your capacity to be in non-ordinary states of consciousness, one step at a time, in predictable settings. The next question is where and with whom you will have your experience. The environment in which you have your journey matters as much as the substance itself.

CHAPTER 3
Choosing Your Setting

Like all butterflies, the tiger-winged monarch begins as a caterpillar. After two weeks spent eating a small mountain of milkweed leaves, the caterpillar sheds her outer skin and forms her protective chrysalis. While inside the golden-green sac, her body essentially dissolves, digesting itself from within. What biologists call imaginal discs—clusters of cells that carry a blueprint for her butterfly body, wings, and antennae—use the dissolved tissue as building material. While dissolving, she has no solid identity or form. She is temporarily vulnerable to predators and heavy rain or wind. Whether she becomes a butterfly depends on the chrysalis that protects her; this delicate yet enduring shell keeps her secure until she emerges black and orange, shimmering in her radiance.

Like the transforming butterfly, when you ingest a psychedelic substance, your psychological defenses are temporarily dismantled, making you highly sensitive to your environment. Each setting has its own benefits and risks. Understanding the range empowers you to advocate for what you need. Options include asking a friend to sit with you, joining a ceremony, hiring a trained guide, or seeking treatment in a state-approved healing center. As you read this chapter, think about who and what you want to be present. Do you want to be in a cozy living room, at a retreat center in the rainforest, in a white-walled clinic, outside in nature, or at a group ceremony surrounded by new people?

Why Your Surroundings Matter

Your brain is continuously processing sensory and social cues, filtering most of them out so you can function. Psychedelics temporarily remove many of those filters. Suddenly, everything your brain usually dismisses as background noise—the texture of the couch, the tone of someone's voice, the quality of light in the room—becomes amplified and potentially meaningful. Your brain is taking in the same information it always does, but without its usual ability to sort signal from noise. This is why your physical space and the people in it matter so much during a psychedelic experience. You're responding to the same environmental cues you always do, just with your filtering system temporarily offline.

During a psychedelic experience, the boundary between self and other can dissolve. Suddenly, everything around you becomes an intimate part of your experience: the decorations on the walls, the sleeping cat, the guitar music, your guide. You want to make sure your environment is the protective chrysalis you need it to be.

This understanding isn't new. While there was plenty of recreational exploration happening in the United States during the 1950s and 1960s, early psychedelic researchers were quick to acknowledge the importance of both set (preparation and intentions) and setting.[1] While this concept got popularized in the 1960s, it goes back even further to the French hashish smokers of the mid-1800s. The poet Charles Baudelaire wrote that an experience of smoking hashish would turn out well if the setting was well-prepared: "if you find yourself in the right environment, such as a picturesque landscape or an apartment that has been decorated artistically, and if you can also hope for a little music."[2] However, the principle is more ancient than that. Cultures around the world have long recognized that ceremonies benefit from intentional settings—specific locations chosen for their proximity to rivers, high bluffs, or mountains and visited at certain times of year.

DO YOU WANT TO BE INSIDE OR OUTSIDE?

One consideration that applies to all settings is whether you want to journey indoors or outdoors. An indoor setting offers containment and boundaries; it's predictable and comfortable. Knowing you can open and close the windows, control the climate, and go to the bathroom with the door closed offers a certain reassurance. Yet, when in an expanded state, indoor environments, especially clinical settings, can feel contrived or sterile.

Alternatively, imagine sitting under an endless blue sky, gazing up into towering pine trees as sunlight streams through, or watching the rising full moon on the horizon. Having a journey in the grand temple that is the natural world can be sublime, as it becomes alive in ways that indoor spaces simply can't match. Yet being outside is unpredictable. A storm can blow in, ants can move in on your spot, or a group of six friends and their dogs can show up across the lake, set up camping chairs, and turn on the '80s rock.

Still, if you can find a private location where you won't be disturbed, during a favorable season, there is nothing like being in the natural elements while you are wide open. A cool wind, birdsong, or the sound of the creek all become part of your journey. The ideal setting would offer the option to be quietly inside, away from the elements, or to be outside to sit on the earth or among the trees, with an easy way to move between them.

Settings for a Psychedelic Experience

FESTIVAL AND PUBLIC SETTINGS

It's a natural impulse to want to change your state of consciousness, whether for play and connection or simply to release the cares of the world at the end of the week. At a weekend music festival, as the sun sets, you might place a small paper square of LSD on your tongue and enjoy a night of exuberant dancing, wandering from stage to stage, mesmerized by hypnotic light shows timed to the music. There is an indescribable wonder in joining an ocean of fellow humans whose consciousness is expanded, and an exhilarating unpredictability to the spontaneous group journey.

However, the dose really matters here. As many experienced journeyers will caution, taking a hefty dose of any psychoactive substance with minimal preparation in an unpredictable public setting is a high-risk gamble. Becoming separated from your friends, wandering disoriented through the night, or navigating a sweaty crowd of intoxicated strangers can quickly become overwhelming or even dangerous. If emotionally painful memories come up, it can be hard to find reassurance on the fly.

But with an appropriate dose for your experience level—start low!—and a basic plan so you know where your friends are and have a set meeting spot, impromptu journeys can be both fun and nourishing. One caution: If you are looking to get substances at festivals, there is no way to know what you are getting unless on-site drug testing is available.

SELF-GUIDED SOLO JOURNEY

Intentional solo journeys take place in a prepared environment, at your home or in nature, and involve more preparation than recreational experiences. It's tempting to journey in the comfort of your bedroom, relaxing in a quiet familiar setting. But journeying alone means navigating whatever arises without support. If you get into rough psychological territory, do you feel able to work with it? Even if you have someone you can call, talking on the phone offers limited support. It may be better to have someone at home with you who can supervise your safety and be available should you need them. A great way to give yourself an extra layer of support is to schedule an integration session for a few days after your journey.

JOURNEYING WITH FRIENDS

Small group journeys with friends offer more support than solo experiences. For example, while camped beside a river, you and a few close friends each take two grams of mushrooms. Perhaps you've planned this night for weeks, and now, sitting beside a snapping fire, you watch shadows dance on pine trees while sharing childhood stories punctuated by long periods of peaceful silence. You feel at ease in the woods with your friends, far from the bustle of city life, and smile at having prepared so thoughtfully for this experience. Having friends by your side is more supportive than journeying with mushrooms alone. However, if everyone is sinking into their own journey and things get rocky for one person, it can be hard for the group. Consider having one person take a lower dose so they can stay available for unanticipated needs. Alternatively, have someone nearby on call if needed.

HAVING A SOBER SITTER

You may want both support and privacy for your inward dive, so you ask a friend or acquaintance to sit with you and keep you safe throughout your journey. Having a sober partner or friend by your side who is fully attentive to you can be bonding for both of you.

If you go this route, make sure you choose someone emotionally stable and trustworthy, ideally with personal experience. Your sitter may offer to help you set up an altar, read a prayer or a poem, or sing to you.

However, an untrained sitter may not know what to do if you become frightened or overwhelmed. Because of the depth of vulnerability that can open up, you may cry, need to scream, confess something from your past, or talk for hours about how frustrated you are with your mother or how much you love your dog. This can ask a lot of a friend or acquaintance if you don't already share a deep bond.

It's good to discuss boundaries, the kind of support you want, and emergency protocols beforehand. I do not recommend that first-time journeyers start with an untrained sitter.

GROUP CEREMONIES

Another option is to join a group ceremony centered around a shared spiritual practice or intention. After hearing about ayahuasca ceremonies for years, you finally decide to join one led by a facilitator visiting from South America. After following preparation guidance for a week, you arrive with your intention, ready to meet this legendary plant teacher in the presence of friends or strangers. With the support of a facilitator and their assistants, you may laugh and cry, often bonding with your fellow participants after only a few days together.

Group ceremonies take many forms, each shaped by the traditions and intentions of those gathering. Some are plant-medicine church events where an ordained minister leads congregants through a sacramental experience. Others are led by healers who travel from abroad to guide participants through ayahuasca or huachuma ceremonies rooted in their ancestral practices. You can find Black medicine circles that come together to sing and pray, Buddhist sanghas that take small amounts of mushrooms before meditating together, and Christian communities that gather to read scripture with the enhancement of their chosen sacrament. Groups of climate activists come together to take medicine, grieve together, and restore themselves before returning to the front lines.

You'll typically join three to twelve other people—although some ceremonies include upward of thirty participants—guided by one or two facilitators with the support of assistants. Group ceremonies range from highly structured to freeform; some require you to sit up all night, while others allow dancing and lying down. Ask about the ceremony's structure beforehand so you know what you are committing to.

In group ceremonies, individual attention is limited, especially in larger gatherings. Assistants are there mainly for practical needs—providing water, adjusting blankets, and helping you to the bathroom. If you are struggling, there might not be anyone available to support you directly. For this reason, group ceremonies may not be ideal for your first psychedelic experience. You'll be navigating both a new state of consciousness and the energy of multiple people.

If you want to attend a ceremony hosted by a plant-medicine church, they may ask you to sign a liability waiver or become a member. Some have an official federal exemption to use an otherwise prohibited substance as a sacrament with their congregants.[3] However, many operate without official exemption, putting them in a legal gray area, even if they host events in a city that has decriminalized their chosen sacrament. If legal risk matters to you, ask questions beforehand to understand what you're signing up for.

Some people opt for group ceremonies because they are more affordable than working with an individual guide. While that's totally understandable, if you feel individual work would be a better fit, first try to find a guide who offers low-fee sessions. If you have a trauma history, it's recommended to have a handful of experiences with personal support before joining a ceremony.

WORKING WITH A TRAINED GUIDE

Many people find they prefer individual support for their journeys, especially if they are new or want to dive into personal healing. If this describes you, consider seeking a trained psychedelic guide—someone who has completed a training program or extended apprenticeship with an experienced teacher.

In contrast to a sitter, a trained guide will bring more experience, having accompanied many psychedelic sessions. They are often better equipped to support you throughout the entire arc of your journey. Your experience will be tailored to you, taking place in a therapy office, a home, or a yurt in the forest. You'll be alone with your guide, though they may bring an assistant. You might go home at the end of the day, or stay overnight, or even for a few days.

A guide should take the time to get to know your history, usually through a series of pre-journey meetings or video calls, and should lead you through your mental and logistical preparation. During your journey, they serve as your attentive guardian, creating the structure for the day and often providing the music and the medicine, although some guides ask you to bring your own. They will support your aftercare over the integration weeks following your journey.

Many trained guides also have training as doctors, nurses, therapists, or life coaches. Others are ordained clergy, herbalists, or bodyworkers, or have spent years apprenticing with teachers trained in traditional healing lineages. Their background and training will influence their worldview about how psychedelic medicines heal, and their worldview will influence how they interact with you.

A trained guide is considered "underground" if they don't work in a legal or regulated setting. The exception includes locations like Colorado, where psilocybin, psilocin, DMT, ibogaine, and mescaline (excluding peyote) have been decriminalized, as long as there is no direct payment for the medicine itself. The substances must be gifted or shared, and facilitators can share medicine with anyone "who is twenty-one years of age or older within the context of counseling, spiritual guidance, beneficial community-based use and healing, supported use, or related services."[4] The next chapter dives deeper into the nuances of working with a guide.

PSYCHEDELIC RETREAT CENTERS

Picture an open-air building with a woven thatched roof, exposed beams, skylight windows, and vegetarian food served on long wooden tables. When you want an experience that isn't available or legal in your home country or are looking for a psychedelic vacation, your options include psilocybin mushroom journeys in Jamaica or the Netherlands, ibogaine treatment in Mexico, or ayahuasca ceremonies in Central or South America.

Psychedelic healing retreats often include joining a group of seekers from around the world and spending a week together sharing group ceremonies or having individual journeys alongside one another. They typically feed you, give you a place to sleep, and sometimes provide therapeutic support. The staff usually includes facilitators and assistants, cooks, and housekeepers. Some retreats offer luxury, while others provide simpler accommodations.

It's good to do your research anytime you travel to a new country, and especially if you're considering a retreat where you will be taking mind-altering substances with new people. Some centers are run by seasoned facilitators who work respectfully with local communities, while others are run by profit-driven entrepreneurs who exploit them. It's hard to gauge a retreat center's quality and integrity from its website photos and testimonials. Consider searching for reviews online or requesting a conversation with one or two past participants.

PSILOCYBIN TREATMENT CENTERS

In Oregon and Colorado, there are legal psilocybin treatment centers where you can work with a licensed facilitator for individual or group journeys. If predictability and formal oversight matter to you, this structure offers reassurance that unregulated settings can't. Regulations make these treatment centers safer in practical ways: The medicine is lab-tested for potency, rules define how facilitators can interact with you, and there's a formal process if something goes wrong.

Some treatment centers are deluxe and others are simple clinics. You'll typically journey in a private room with the door closed, knowing others are on their own journeys down the hallway. Facilitators charge fees similar to underground guides, and sometimes offer scholarships or sliding-scale options.

All facilitators complete a state-approved training program and pass the licensing test.[5] However, being licensed doesn't mean they are therapeutically trained beyond the required 120 hours. In Colorado, you can choose between clinical facilitators with mental health credentials and nonclinical facilitators who work with lower-risk participants.

Facilitator training programs vary in approach and rigor, and facilitators' personal experience ranges widely. I've met facilitators whose only psilocybin experience was their required group practicum, while others have years of professional and personal experience. Ask about your facilitator's background, training, and personal experience before committing.

KETAMINE CLINICS

Ketamine is a popular treatment for depression, anxiety, and chronic pain. The benefits of receiving ketamine at a clinic include medical supervision, legal access, and possibly insurance reimbursement. You'll likely sit in a reclining chair while receiving the substance as a nasal spray, through an IV, or as an intramuscular injection. A nurse or doctor will monitor your vital signs throughout the session, which usually lasts about an hour. Some clinics, especially those offering injections, provide eye masks and headphones with music and have someone stay with you the entire time. Others may give you the medicine and leave you alone in a private or group treatment room.

The quality and approach of ketamine clinics vary widely. Some are run by psychiatrists or therapists who help you prepare and offer integration sessions afterward. Others are run by anesthesiologists who see ketamine as a medical treatment: You'll get medical supervision but minimal therapeutic support. You may get symptom relief without a transformative experience.

If you're considering a ketamine treatment at a clinic, ask questions like: Do you believe ketamine can offer psychological healing, or just symptom reduction? Do you offer preparation or integration support? Will someone stay with me during my entire session? What's your approach to dosing?

CLINICAL TRIALS

Although they might not offer the most idyllic setting, clinical trials provide a structured environment where you'll be attended to by licensed doctors, nurses, therapists, or other mental health professionals. This is a suitable setting for people who need predictability and want the highest level of physical safety.

You will likely be in a hospital or clinic, in a carefully crafted environment that includes a couch, a blindfold, a blood pressure monitor, and tasteful innocuous art on the walls. Often two facilitators will be with you, and the psychedelic experience, usually called a "dosing session," is often video recorded.

Clinical trials offer free treatment and often provide compensation to cover your time and travel costs. From intake to completion, your involvement could span weeks to many months. Most trials involve a control group, meaning you may spend months preparing only to receive a placebo. However, most psychedelic clinical trials eventually offer the active medicine to everyone, though this could require waiting additional months.

If you are considering joining a clinical trial, pay attention to the research focus. Is it a neuroscience study where they give you LSD and scan your brain with a functional MRI machine? Or are the researchers studying the combination of psilocybin with a specific therapeutic approach? If you have a trauma history, make sure the trial will be a good fit for your needs. Most clinical trials have strict eligibility requirements, and if you have a complex medical or psychiatric background, you may not qualify. There are online resources to search for clinical trials worldwide.[6]

What Setting Will Hold You Best?

Now that you understand your options, take time to reflect honestly on your needs. What will help you relax and serve your healing? How much support do you actually need? How much privacy? What level of risk are you willing to tolerate physically, psychologically, or legally? No facilitator, guide, or expert knows the answers to these questions better than you do. If you're uncertain, you might need more time to think it through or to have more conversations with people about their experiences. Choosing to wait until you have all the information you need to make a comfortable choice is wise. There is no universally "best" setting. What is best is whatever is most suitable for you at this time in your life.

CHAPTER 4

Working with a Psychedelic Guide

The healing guide's role is ancient. Historically referred to as shamans, curanderos (traditional healers), or "medicine people," guides have fulfilled an essential social role for thousands of years across many cultures.[1] These are individuals trained to accompany you into non-ordinary states of consciousness for healing or exploration. They might help you enter these states by guiding you through a multiday fast or a drumming journey. They are also trained to assist you if you want to ingest psychoactive plants or fungi as part of your healing path.

Traditionally trained healing guides are often born into their vocation as family heirs to a lineage. Others come to their paths after recovery from a personal illness or after surviving a tragedy that inspires them to help others. Many traditionally trained guides have spent decades by their teacher's side learning the healing arts through observation and osmosis while accumulating their own personal experience.

Most contemporary psychedelic guides are not traditional shamans, though some have spent years learning from them or other spiritual teachers around the world. The majority are therapists or coaches, although some may be doctors, nurses, or clergy who have sought out additional training in psychedelic facilitation.

Who you choose as a guide will be one of the most consequential decisions you'll make. This person will witness you at your most vulnerable, sit beside you through what might feel like death and rebirth, and help you make sense of what you saw and felt. Yet most people spend less time vetting their guide than they do researching a new car. The person by your side will have a marked impact on your experience. Learn about their background and their views of the world. You want to check out who they really are.

While you can embark on a psychedelic journey without direct support—many have, and many do—the presence of a trusted guide can help you relax into unfamiliar territory, soften into your grief, or move through painful memories. They are there by your side, no matter what arises, and they provide an anchor when you need one. They are there to help you land at the end of your journey by feeding you fruit and tea as you slowly return from the depths. There is something innately human in wanting steady, caring support as you move through intense shifts in consciousness.

To help you understand your options, I'll describe the difference between licensed facilitators at state-approved healing centers, group facilitators, and trained underground guides. I will describe the services a psychedelic guide typically offers, why you might consider working with one, and suggest how to get clear about what you are looking for. I've also created a comprehensive list of questions to use as a map when meeting a potential guide, which you can find in appendix B.

What Does a Psychedelic Guide Do?

The psychedelic guide's job combines the skills of a therapist (understanding human behavior and building rapport), a pharmacist (knowing dosage and which medicines don't mix safely), and a midwife (calmly supporting a healing process that can be as intense as childbirth). They're also there to minimize unnecessary stress, manage expectations and disappointments, and prevent emergencies.

A guide's work typically unfolds in four phases: assessment, preparation, the journey itself, and integration.

CARE BEGINS WITH INTAKE

The psychedelic guide's first job is to keep you safe. This begins with a medical screening and intake process to assess whether, based on your health conditions, history, and current life circumstances, a psychedelic journey is appropriate for you right now. If they have any concerns or if your medical situation is complicated in any way, they should refer you to a medical provider knowledgeable about psychedelics for further consultation. A guide should never advise you to stop or taper off your medications. They should always defer to your prescriber, who can help you weigh the risks and benefits of stopping a medication and help you do it safely. Part of the intake is assessing whether they're equipped to work with you or should refer you to someone better suited to your needs.

PREPARING BODY, MIND, AND HEART

If it's a good fit—that is, you feel safe with them, and it seems like they understand you—then you're ready to proceed. Your guide will help you prepare for your journey, including clarifying your intentions. They should remind you of what to avoid the week before (certain foods, other substances, stressful situations), what to bring, whether you will need to be dropped off, and other logistical details. It's their job to provide a safe, comfortable journey space for you, or help you find one ahead of time and adapt it to your needs.

Your guide should explain which medicine they think is best for you and discuss dosage beforehand. They should test every new batch of medicine to ensure purity and confirm potency. This is necessary so they can determine precisely how much to give you, based on your level of experience and intentions. Ideally, your guide will have a cautious approach to dosing. Remember: You can always take more, but it's hard to take less.

SITTING BY YOUR SIDE

During your journey, a guide's role shifts to being your guardian, someone you will trust to manage the outer world so you can explore your inner world. It's their job to welcome you into a supportive environment, having prepared the room and attended to little details, such as ensuring you have plenty of blankets and that your water bottle is nearby. They will draw the curtains, feed the fire, and keep the candles lit. They will whistle, sing, or play recorded music, maintaining a steady flow of melody for your attention to follow, and when needed, slowly guide you to the bathroom.

An experienced guide will stay close enough to hear and see you without crowding your space. They will take notes throughout—recording what you say, the gestures you make, the emotions that arise, and the memories that emerge. Because a psychedelic experience can reveal what needs attention in your life and deliver unexpected insights, having a record of everything you speak out loud or express nonverbally becomes invaluable later.

If you find yourself in daunting territory, a skillful guide should be able to discern whether you are courageously meeting your fear or stuck in a repeating loop and approaching overwhelm. They should know when to remind you that they are right there beside you, or offer you a hand to hold.

HELPING YOU RETURN

Your guide should help you land at the end of the day, ensure you are hydrated and fed, and have a safe ride home and a warm place to sleep. They should check on you over the next few days and make sure you are doing okay. When it comes time to meet for an integration session and discuss your journey, they should have taken time to reflect on your experience so they are ready to debrief with you. If any concerning issues arise after your journey—if you feel disoriented, can't sleep, or feel depressed or highly emotional for more than a few days—they should stay in close contact and connect you with additional support.

TWO APPROACHES: DIRECTIVE AND NONDIRECTIVE

Most guides work in one of two styles or land somewhere in between.

Nondirective: If they are trained as a clinical therapist or in the lineage of Holotropic Breathwork, as many guides are, they will minimize interventions and focus on providing a steady, loving presence. Sometimes this is called "non-doing." Instead of following any agenda, they will follow your own inner healing intelligence. A guide who prefers this nondirective approach will often reflect your questions back to you instead of giving you their opinion or advice, helping you explore your questions on your own terms. They may be more proactive about discussing boundaries and consent. If they follow standard psychotherapeutic guidelines on ethics, it will often make for a simpler, more straightforward relationship.

Directive: Other guides who have trained as healers or curanderos or apprenticed with traditional teachers may bring a worldview that could be considered more shamanic. They might use more interventions, such as bodywork or energy healing, musical instruments, songs, or prayers. They may use stones, smoke, feathers, scented essential oils, or gongs. Their underlying philosophy differs from the nondirective approach. As one *ayahuasquero* explained to me, the shamanic approach can be summed up simply: "Bad stuff out, good stuff in." They often focus on extracting what doesn't belong and calling in what does.

Guides trained in shamanic approaches may have been trained to see things others can't and to address issues in ways that therapists can't comprehend. Because they often become more involved, greater skill and sensitivity are needed. When stronger interventions are attempted without proper training and careful conduct, there can be greater potential for harm.

If they have only experienced one style, they might not understand the other and may even have a strong bias. Many guides blend these two styles or tend toward one or the other, depending on the situation. Consider which style would be most comfortable for you.

PROFESSIONAL CONDUCT OF A PSYCHEDELIC GUIDE

During all sessions and especially during a journey, your guide should:

- Be on time or let you know if they are running late.
- Be prepared, present, and settled.
- Be close enough to hear your words, see your movements, and talk with you, but far away enough to allow you your personal space.

- Give you their full, calm attention.
- Take notes during your journey.
- Respect your requests to lower the volume or turn the music off.
- Honor your boundaries.
- Tell you when they are leaving the room for any reason and confirm that you are okay being left alone for a few minutes. They should let you know when they have returned, either verbally or through another method.
- Feed you after the session. Your guide should either have food on hand or have told you to bring your own.
- Demonstrate respect, self-care, and self-reflection.

The Relationship Matters

Regardless of style or technique, trust matters most in a healing relationship. Studies repeatedly show that the quality of your relationship and sense of connection with your facilitator are among the strongest predictors of a successful outcome.[2] Trust isn't instant—it often takes time to grow. If a guide is not willing to meet with you a few times before a psychedelic session to get to know each other, you might reconsider whether they are right for you. Hurrying into an experience with minimal preparation may save time and money, but it will cost you in other ways.

During your initial meetings with a potential guide, whether in person or virtually, pay attention to the quality of your connection. Do you feel a natural ease growing between you? If not, once the medicine takes effect, your unease can intensify. This is especially true if you know you are someone who really needs to feel safe around people. Instead of focusing on your own experience, you may find yourself watching your guide, continually checking whether they're present with you. This preoccupation can pull your attention away from yourself, where it should be, and toward your guide, keeping you stuck in ordinary awareness rather than deepening.

Think of it this way: Would you trust this person to take you on an icy high-altitude mountain climb? I don't recommend moving forward with a guided psychedelic session until you feel a solid sense of trust, even if it requires meeting multiple times beforehand. It takes as long as it takes.

What to Look for in a Psychedelic Guide

SEASONED AND STEADY

What specific qualities and characteristics should guide your search? The number-one requirement for a guide is familiarity with the dynamic nature of the psychedelic territory. There's no substitute for personal experience—the more, the better. They also need to have received formal training or apprenticed with an experienced guide. If someone has only studied theories of consciousness and read psychedelic research, they aren't ready to guide anyone.

The psychedelic experience is multidimensional and can include unpredictable physical, emotional, and transpersonal phenomena. Your lips can tremble, your legs might shake, your face may flush. One minute you might feel like you're twelve years old; the next moment you might feel like a baby. You can experience sublime beauty and sink into the depths of long-repressed emotions, sometimes in the span of just ten minutes. You want your guide to have traveled these realms themselves—extensively—so nothing you experience will surprise or unsettle them.

When the medicine takes effect, the body can release in dramatic and unexpected ways: through sweat, mucus, tears, or sobs. One seasoned guide told me that at the climax of a high-dose LSD journey, he smelled the unmistakable odor of brandy coming from the pores of a client who had been sober for ten years. A skilled guide with enough personal experience, at least of comparable intensity, will not be startled by any of this.

Your guide's quality of presence matters too. Humans naturally pick up on each other's emotional states, so finding someone whose nervous system is as steady or steadier than yours will mean they can help you stabilize if the waves get choppy. On the other hand, if your guide is distracted or ungrounded, you'll likely sense it—and it could increase your own anxiety. If they remain calm, present, and caring, you'll be able to exhale and let go. Because everything during a psychedelic journey is intensified, their emotional state, tone of voice, and choice of words create an atmosphere that can directly affect your experience. Their warm and welcoming companionship will help you relax, while their steady, grounded presence can help you stabilize when things get hard.

IDENTITY, EXPERIENCE, AND EXPERTISE

Choosing a psychedelic guide is similar to selecting a therapist. On a practical level, you want to find someone whose location, availability, and fees make sense for your life. You also want someone with enough life experience to understand what you're going through.

Working with someone who has dealt with similar life struggles or shares aspects of your identity can create an immediate connection. If you are newly retired and navigating life without the daily anchor of work, you may want to find someone who can relate to your situation. If you are a person of color, you may want a guide who shares your background or understands the nuances of your life experience. If you are exploring issues around your sexuality or gender, consider finding someone who has walked a similar path.

Consider whether you want specific expertise. Are you three decades into a marriage that is flailing? Look for someone who focuses on sexual or intimacy issues. Do you have a complex medical history, autoimmune issues, or take medications? Look for someone medically trained. Are you struggling with residual anxiety after cancer or facing a terminal diagnosis? You may want a guide who has supported someone through serious illness or has been through it themselves. To work with unresolved trauma, look for a guide who is trauma-trained. The same goes for addiction, childhood neglect or abuse, or the recent loss of a parent or loved one: You want to seek out a guide with relevant training and experience.

Consider the personal qualities you'd appreciate most. Do you prefer someone who is more analytical or emotionally intuitive? Someone with shamanic training and years of apprenticeship, or someone clinically trained as a therapist? Someone who understands the creative process or the pressures of the business world? A guide who speaks your native language or shares your spiritual tradition?

WORKING SOLO OR WITH A COFACILITATOR

In many traditional settings, a primary guide often has an assistant or apprentice by their side, taking care of practical matters so they can focus on the healing work itself. There are benefits to having at least two facilitators, and most clinical trials have been designed with this in mind.[3] Accompanying someone throughout a psychedelic journey can include hours of attentive listening, note-taking, and handholding. With two facilitators, they can share responsibilities, take breaks, and be better protected against ethical missteps that can occur in the intimacy of a one-on-one setting.

Others choose to work solo because they prefer the intimacy of one-on-one work. Working alone with a guide can bring up strong feelings—sometimes toward the guide themselves. When a guide handles this well, it can deepen the healing. When they don't, it gets messy. You can ask a potential guide whether they have an assistant and why they've chosen their approach, and consider their rationale in your decision-making.

LAYERS OF SUPPORT

Your guide needs their own support system to support you effectively. Best practice in the underground is that if a guide has been working with clients for less than five years, they should be getting regular mentorship or supervision from a more senior practitioner. Anyone guiding others with psychedelics should have ongoing support, at least regular peer consultation, throughout their career. Because psychedelic work is so intense, it's easy for a guide to get caught up in complicated dynamics (more on that in chapter 10). They should have a supervisor or mentor who offers an outside perspective and can help them through complex situations. Of course, whether they have this support in place is not your responsibility, but you can ask them about it. Their response will speak to their commitment to ethical practice.

Practical Considerations

TRAINING AND CREDENTIALS

The landscape of guides includes people working in regulated settings, religious contexts, medical practices, and underground. Their training and legal positioning vary widely. Understanding these distinctions can help you decide what matters most to you.

Licensed facilitator: In Oregon, Colorado, and New Mexico, you can work with state-licensed psilocybin facilitators who have completed required training programs and comply with state regulations. Because they are licensed, there is a place to file a complaint if needed, which offers greater protection.

Plant-medicine church ministers: Some guides work as ordained ministers within plant-medicine churches. As mentioned, a handful of these churches hold federal exemptions allowing them to legally serve otherwise prohibited medicines during ceremonies. If you are considering working with a minister-guide from a plant-medicine church, you can ask whether their church has a legal exemption, and if not, what their relationship to the law is. Also ask whether the church has an ethical code of conduct or a governing board that handles complaints.

Ketamine providers: Ketamine is legally available through clinics and can be prescribed by doctors or nurses to take with a therapist or for at-home use. While there is no official ketamine training license, there are solid trainings available. You can ask what kind of training your ketamine therapist received and check it out. Was it a weekend workshop or a six-month program? Were they educated by seasoned ketamine therapists and clinicians connected with a reputable healing center or ketamine clinic? Did they learn through apprenticeship from a seasoned psychedelic therapist? Or were they trained by a medical doctor who taught them how to administer ketamine safely, but included little to no therapeutic understanding?

Trained guide: The majority of psychedelic guides in the United States are working without licenses or state approval. Many trainings exist, from year-long underground guide trainings to three-day-long "psychedelic coaching programs." Others learn through multiyear apprenticeships, sitting by their teacher's side. These have no official approval or oversight and do not offer a state-recognized license or certification. Training is essential, and some of these programs are comprehensive, but you want to ask questions to learn what their training included.

And while psilocybin has been decriminalized in many cities across the United States, as mentioned, local decriminalization doesn't mean facilitation services are legal. Regardless of license status or credentials, it's wise to ask about training, supervision, and how they deal with ethical dilemmas.

Ceremony leaders: Group ceremonies are often led by trained guides or ceremonialists who have apprenticed in a traditional healing lineage. Leading group ceremonies is different from individual work and requires specific skills. Beware of ceremony leaders who have attended ceremonies as a participant but haven't actually been trained. Traveling to other countries to participate in ceremonies is a wonderful thing, but it does not train you to lead groups. Ask ceremony leaders who their teachers are and what their training or apprenticeship consisted of.

FEES

Many people are initially surprised when they hear a guide's fee. Some charge hourly for preparation, integration, and journey sessions, with costs varying by location and experience. Fees commonly range from $100 to $250 per hour. Others charge a flat rate for the "package," typically $1,000 or more, regardless of the number of hours spent on your journey day, which removes pressure to wrap up by a specific time. Remember that if they are a licensed therapist or experienced coach, they are spending the entire day with you rather than seeing multiple clients. Many guides offer sliding-scale options, and newer guides are likely to charge lower fees, making the work more affordable. It's always worth asking if they can work with your budget.

HOW MANY SESSIONS AND HOW OFTEN

Do you want to work with a guide just once or a few times, or are you hoping to develop a relationship over time? Guides typically require one to three preparation sessions before the journey day, followed by one to three integration sessions. A short-term commitment lets you decide whether you want to keep working with them. However, healing typically happens over time, partly because of the increasing trust you build with your guide. For this reason, many guides offer psychedelic sessions as part of longer-term work. Aim for at least three journeys with preparation and integration spread over time if you want to understand what guided work can offer.

In my experience, allowing six to twelve weeks between journeys provides enough time to integrate your previous experience. Fewer than six weeks may not give you enough time to fully integrate your last experience. Exceptions include ceremonies happening over two to three consecutive days or medicines like ketamine, which can work well when sessions are scheduled closer together.

Finding a Guide

Modern marketing has flooded into all tributaries of the healing field, and psychedelic guide work is no exception. Visually stunning websites abound. Look beyond the polished branding and expand your search beyond social media. A skilled guide doesn't need to oversell themselves; their competence shows through in how they answer your questions and the substance of their training.

If someone offers services as a certified psychedelic guide, coach, or healer, examine their training. What did it include, how long was it, and who were their teachers? Guides trained through apprenticeship may not share their teachers' names publicly, preferring to wait until they trust you. However, you can ask general questions about their lineage and how many years they spent training. Again, beware of ceremony leaders who have only attended a handful of ceremonies abroad and haven't actually completed a thorough apprenticeship. While spending five-plus years in an academic institution studying psychology or obtaining a medical degree is substantial training, it doesn't guarantee skill in guiding people through psychedelic experiences.

When seeking a referral, it's best to go with good old-fashioned word of mouth when you can. Ask people in your community if they can recommend anyone. Attend psychedelic conferences or look for psychedelic integration circles in your area or online. Oregon and Colorado maintain public lists of licensed psilocybin facilitators, and you can call licensed service centers (called healing centers in Colorado) to learn more about their practitioners, then reach out for a conversation.

Remember to bring intuition to your search; watch for signs, and trust your gut. If you are coincidentally referred to the same guide twice, it may be worth exploring, even if their age or gender doesn't match what you thought you wanted. The healing path isn't always rational, and unexpected connections often point the way.

HAVE A CONVERSATION

Before committing to working with a psychedelic guide, schedule an initial meeting—either in person, by phone, or video call. This conversation allows you to assess their depth of training, personal experience, and ethical framework while giving you both a chance to gauge whether you'll work well together. Just as you would carefully vet a surgeon before undergoing a major procedure, you need to ask thoughtful questions to ensure you're choosing a guide with both competence and integrity.

The basic topics you want to ask about include their availability and fee, their background and training, how they approach safety and screening, which substances they use, and where sessions take place. You also want to ask about touch and consent, how they approach integration, and their approach to ethics. You can also ask questions specific to your identity and intentions.

For a complete list of questions, go to my list of "Questions to Ask Before Choosing a Psychedelic Guide" in appendix B.

AFTER YOU MEET

Pay attention to how you felt during your conversation. Did the guide listen well? Did they ask thoughtful questions about you and your intentions? Did they answer your concerns directly and thoroughly? Did they seem more interested in whether this work is right for you, or in signing you up? A responsible guide will assess whether they can genuinely serve you, not just whether you can pay their fee.

Did you feel comfortable asking direct questions, or did you feel pressured to stay polite and avoid topics that might create tension? A good guide will welcome your questions, including ones about their training, boundaries, or past complaints. If someone becomes defensive when you ask about their training or if they have had any formal complaints filed against them, that tells you what you need to know.

If something feels off during your initial conversation, even if you can't articulate what it is, pay attention to that. At the same time, some nervousness is normal when meeting someone with whom you are considering such intimate work. Did you feel increasingly at ease as the conversation progressed, or did your discomfort persist or intensify?

Do you feel confident in this person's training and approach? Do their answers to your questions satisfy you, or are there lingering concerns? If you notice yourself making excuses for red flags or talking yourself out of legitimate concerns, pause and reconsider. If you don't feel comfortable moving forward, you can ask them if they are willing to give you another referral based on what exactly you are looking for. You don't owe anyone your trust when it comes to your safety.

Strong communication skills, the ability to sense what you need, and clear boundaries are essential for a good relationship with your guide. If those aren't present, your relationship is more likely to break down as the work gets harder. I've dedicated chapter 10 to navigating the relationship with a psychedelic guide, including safety concerns and what to do when problems arise.

The Choice Is Yours

Taking this much time to find the right guide may seem excessive, but I'd say it's appropriate given what you're entrusting them with. The truth is, if you want to explore guided work, who you choose to work with is one of the most important decisions you will make. A skilled guide creates the conditions for healing by managing both the practical and energetic environment, allowing the part of you that usually stays vigilant to rest so you can explore more freely. Their training, experience, and presence directly shape your experience and ensure your safety.

Whether or not you decide to work with a guide is ultimately your choice. Some people find that having skilled support makes all the difference in their healing. Others prefer to journey on their own, with trusted friends, or in community. All paths can work.

Even if you decide not to work with a guide, understanding what good guidance looks like can help you create better conditions for yourself or support friends and family who are exploring this path. And if you do choose guided work, it is absolutely worth your time to find just the right person; it will make all the difference.

CHAPTER 5
Choosing Your Medicine

A molecule is a molecule is a molecule. The question is not "Is it natural?" but rather "What does it do?"

—ALEXANDER SHULGIN

Each psychedelic medicine has its own intelligence. Many people who work with these medicines come to experience this intelligence as a distinct personality or spirit.

When deciding which medicine you want to "meet," think about what you are coming to your journey for. If you think of it as a teacher, what do you want to learn? If you think of the medicine as a catalyst, what do you want to bring into being? If you think of it as a gateway, a gateway to what? Given what you already know, which medicine do you feel drawn to connect with? Of course, knowing what's legal and available where you live will also be part of your decision.

To help you explore these questions, I'll cover natural and synthetic medicines as well as sourcing, dosage, and potency. I'll share some unique characteristics of a range of medicines, focusing on the ones you are most likely to be offered by a trained guide, at a healing clinic, or at a ceremony.

However, remember that your experience isn't solely a result of the substance; it's about everything surrounding it. The best outcomes often come for people fortunate enough to have a conducive setting, a clear intention, and the right kind of support alongside a potent medicine.

Natural (Whole-Plant) and Synthetic Medicines

In the world of psychedelics, a distinction is made between whole-plant medicines and lab-made synthetic medicines. Whole-plant medicines are picked, dried, cooked, or made into a liquid extract and are chewed, swallowed, snorted, or smoked. For example, psilocybin mushrooms grow on the earth. You can pick them (after correctly identifying them), eat them fresh, and feel their effects within minutes. Ayahuasca is a combination of two plants, sometimes with added roots, bark, or leaves, that transforms into a powerful psychoactive tea after hours of cooking over the fire. Synthetic substances like LSD, ketamine, and MDMA are made in regulated or clandestine laboratories. The process requires raw chemical ingredients and a chemist who works with precise measurements, temperature, and pH levels. These substances are typically produced as crystalline solids that can be crushed into powder or dissolved into liquid.

Some people are critical of synthetic psychedelic medicines, feeling strongly that consuming whole-plant medicines is superior. My perspective is that they all come from the earth, though some require a more complex alchemical process to become medicine. When it comes to synthetic medicines, the more important questions are: Is it pure? Is it a known substance with years of human use and proof that it's safe?

Sourcing

Many traditions see psychedelic plants and mushrooms as alive and highly absorbent; like sponges, they take in impressions from everything they come into contact with. In a perfect world, you would grow your own medicine or know the person growing or synthesizing it, and ensure they were doing so impeccably.

Years ago in the Amazon, I went into the forest with the head ayahuasquero to gather the plants that would become our ayahuasca. Each time a plant was gathered, he would blow tobacco smoke to make an offering of gratitude for what we took. The next two days were spent in careful quiet preparation and cooking, with more offerings to the plants and spirits of the forest.

As with fine wines, some connoisseurs say they can tell the difference between psychedelic mushrooms found in the wild and those grown indoors. A life-form with its roots deep in the soil, drinking in sun and moonlight, is different from one grown in a sterile laboratory under artificial light. It seems natural that any living being would feel this difference. When medicines are produced in a laboratory, the inputs are more controlled, making the potency more predictable. Either way, you want clean and ethically grown, harvested, or synthesized medicine.

If you are working with a trained guide, they will almost always provide the medicine. You can ask where it comes from, though sometimes this information is kept confidential. Because potency can vary widely in natural medicines, it's always recommended that anyone serving a medicine has ingested the same batch. The exception is at psilocybin service centers, where all mushrooms, extracts, and edibles have been lab-tested for potency. Questions to ask of anyone serving you medicine:

- Where does this medicine come from?
- Who grew it or synthesized it?
- Was it harvested ethically by people being paid fair wages?
- Has it been tested for potency and contaminants?
- Have you tried this particular batch?
- Is it more or less potent than average?

Dosage and Potency

What is there that is not poison? All things are poison and nothing is without poison. Solely the dose determines that a thing is not a poison.

—PARACELSUS

If you are working with a facilitator, they will likely determine your dosage and may invite your input. If you are heading out on a recreational or self-guided journey, you will make this decision yourself. The "heroic dose"—5 grams of dried mushrooms—has been popularized as providing the ultimate psychedelic experience, and many people are eager to jump into a high-dose experience. But the psychological risks are high. There are thresholds after which your experience intensifies quickly. We all want breakthroughs, but why rush?

You can think about psychedelic journeys as rigorous training for your body, heart, and mind. You don't go to the gym and start with hundred-pound weights. You start with the bar and learn the form, then gradually add weight. The same principle applies here: Start low and go slow, building your capacity incrementally. Low-dose journeys are lower risk for accidents or overwhelm and are easier to integrate afterward. As anyone who has had an overwhelmingly strong experience they weren't prepared for will attest, more is not always better. This is especially true if you choose a recreational, self-guided, or sitter-supported journey.

Here are dose levels that apply to most medicines, though the actual amount will vary depending on potency. The intensity of the experience depends on additional factors, including what's going on in your life, how stressed or relaxed you are, and your setting.

Microdose: Also called a subperceptual dose, this is the amount you should barely feel and can take without it affecting your normal daily activities. People take microdoses to increase focus, boost their mood, and enhance creativity.

Minidose: Also called a threshold dose or a museum dose. The idea is that you feel it but can still do some normal activities. You should plan not to drive or work, but some people enjoy this dosage while hiking, cooking, socializing, or practicing yoga or meditation.

Medium dose: This is moving into deeper healing territory. Though some people take this dosage before a concert or party, be careful: Events can be busy and noisy, and you might not want to talk or even walk. Make sure you have a safe place to lie down if you want or need to sink into your internal experience. This is a good amount for sitting in nature or creative activities like playing music or painting. Some people begin to experience visual effects at this threshold, and you may be pulled into an internal journey.

Macrodose: Also known as a therapeutic dose, this is the amount that will give you the experience of full expansion. That is, you move beyond your usual ego-based experience of self as separate from the world. You may not be able to walk or talk, and you really shouldn't. You will likely need help drinking water, going to the bathroom, and staying warm. You should be somewhere safe and protected, ideally with an experienced and sober sitter or a trained guide.

⁂

If you are planning your first journey, you might take an introductory minidose first to get to know the medicine before jumping into a higher dose. You could try 1 gram of mushrooms to get a sense of how it lands in your body and mind. One exception to this guideline is when you're facing a terminal diagnosis. If you might have only one chance to do a high-dose journey and you understand the risks, I recommend taking the dose that gives you the experience you're seeking.

Everyone is different, and though there are general dosage and potency ranges, one person's minidose can be another person's macrodose. Many people are surprised by how taking medicine in a group setting or with a facilitator can intensify the experience. Even if you've taken a particular dosage recreationally before, you may be surprised by how much stronger it becomes when you have prepared well, have a guide sitting beside you, and finally close your eyes.

An experienced guide I know was persuaded by a new client who insisted that hundreds of LSD journeys with friends over the years had prepared him for a high-dose guided session. Soon after the medicine came on, he panicked and tried to run out of the house. He eventually calmed down, and everyone was okay, but he had been mistaken in his confidence.

Meeting the Medicines

CANNABIS: SENSING AND FEELING

Cannabis is a versatile plant that many people use to relax after work, help with sleep, or alleviate physical and emotional pain. I include it here because it's legal in many US states and more and more people are using it in journeys and ceremonies. Cannabis isn't a classic psychedelic and can act as a depressant or stimulant, depending on the strain and potency. However, at a certain dosage threshold, its effects are, without a doubt, psychedelic. If that's how you'd like to approach this medicine, do so with healthy respect and consider all the precautions that apply to classic psychedelics.

Cannabis has two main active ingredients, tetrahydrocannabinol and cannabidiol, known by their acronyms, THC and CBD. Though there are many cannabinoids that all work together, THC is the one that most changes your consciousness. CBD can help calm and settle your nervous system and is often used by people wanting a good night's sleep.

This plant has been used medically and spiritually for over 2,500 years and cultivated for at least 12,000. In Chinese herbal medicine it has been used for centuries, mainly for pain relief. In India it became associated with certain Shaivite sects, and many yogis continue to use it as a sacred sacrament.[1]

Cannabis can be unpredictable. Some people find it relaxing and helpful for PTSD symptoms, while others find it activates anxiety and even paranoia. Its effects depend on the strain and the dose, which can be adjusted puff by puff. One may be enough! As old-timers will tell you, it's much more potent than it used to be.

With edibles, it's best to start low and give them plenty of time to come on before taking more. If they are homemade, you have no way to know their potency. A very experienced friend casually ate waffles made with cannabis butter at a neighbor's house one morning before going on a bike ride along the coast. After an hour, she realized she couldn't go any further. As she told me later, "I ended up on the beach staring at my hands for eight hours. It was a long day, and thank God I had water, but I got a terrible sunburn. I'm staying away from the green butter from now on."

Because cannabis is still illegal at the federal level, safety studies lag behind the commercialization of myriad concentrates, extracts, and other products that have emerged with state-by-state legalization. Many of these products are untested. If you're buying this medicine at a dispensary, look for products with clear labeling that shows THC content. Avoid anything that doesn't specify what's in it or how potent it is. I'd recommend sticking to tinctures, well-labeled gummies, or the dried flowers. If you are new, start with 1 mg of THC and slowly work your way up.

When approached with preparation and respect, a cannabis journey can offer an insightful, often body-centered experience. But approach it with care: This plant is a powerful teacher who can open many dimensions of healing. I've had hundreds of psychedelic experiences, and the two that were most intense and humbling were cannabis journeys. Don't underestimate this plant.

PSILOCYBIN MUSHROOMS: EARTH MEDICINE

Psilocybin mushrooms can be found worldwide, and cave art in northern Africa reaching back seven thousand years depicts what several researchers, including ethnobotanists and mycologists, interpret as psilocybin mushrooms.[2] Similar mushroom imagery appears in ancient carved reliefs, statues, and religious art across Spain, Scotland, Egypt, Greece, India, and Central America—depictions that many scholars believe represent psychoactive species.[3] Mexico has the best-documented continuous tradition of healers who have used sacred mushrooms for centuries. The Mazatec, Zapotec, Mixtec, and other Indigenous groups in the area are the living guardians of this medicine, having kept their ritual practice thriving through generations of colonial suppression.[4]

Clinically, psilocybin has been shown in multiple studies to be effective for treating depression. However, there appears to be a dosage threshold—25 mg—at which most people receive the antidepressant response, the same dosage threshold at which some people report a mystical experience.[5] Once inside your body, psilocybin converts to psilocin, which mimics serotonin by binding to the same receptors. The experience typically lasts around five hours.

Psilocybin mushrooms offer an excellent gateway to introspection and internal work. There's a unique quality to how this medicine feels in the body and psyche; it can soften, melt, and break things down. In nature, mushrooms decompose and detoxify. In the forest, underground fungal networks—called mycelium—connect trees and plants, allowing them to share nutrients. It's as though mushrooms do this within our minds and bodies, making them helpful for processing ancestral trauma and grief. They can open communication and foster connection with ourselves, with each other, and with the greater world. At lower doses, they can be delightful in groups or in ceremony. If you have a mushroom journey, I recommend integration support. This medicine can take you deeper and farther than you can imagine.

AYAHUASCA: VINE OF THE SOULS

For generations, ayahuasca has been used for healing and divination by trained ayahuasqueros and curanderos throughout the Amazon basin of South America. As a sacred medicine it is woven into complex cultural practices and ways of understanding the world that cannot be grasped by simply drinking it. These days, along with the Indigenous and mestizo guides who open their ceremonies to foreigners, there are people of every nationality with varying levels of training offering ayahuasca ceremonies around the world.

Ayahuasca is also known as *yagé* and *Daime*, though the method of preparation and cultural settings differ considerably. It can be intensely introspective, showing you your life's story, but it can also be brilliantly visionary and transpersonal. You can revisit your childhood, travel to other dimensions, and enter different forms of life. Many people encounter ayahuasca's palpable "personality" during a ceremony. The ayahuasca experience can last from four to six hours, but in many ceremonies, you drink the tea multiple times, so it can easily last through the night and into the next morning. Unlike mushrooms or LSD, drinking multiple nights in a row can give you increasingly stronger journeys.

Ayahuasca is unique among psychedelic medicines because it's a combination of two plants and requires preparation. Its active ingredient, DMT, belongs to the same family of classic psychedelics as psilocybin and LSD, which all act on serotonin receptors. However, DMT has a unique mechanism: It's inactive when taken orally because enzymes break it down before it can reach your brain. The genius of ayahuasca is that it combines DMT-containing leaves with the ayahuasca vine, which contains enzyme inhibitors. When cooked into a tea, the combination allows the DMT to survive digestion and reach your brain. This medicinal tea is made from a vine that reaches high into the heavens and a humble leaf that grows close to the ground—the aspiring and the grounding energies combined.

It's invaluable to get integration support after an ayahuasca experience, whether in community or with a therapist or guide. Because of ayahuasca's intensity and wide range of effects, it's not recommended that people with unresolved trauma begin with this medicine. If you are joining an ayahuasca ceremony or traveling to a retreat center that serves this medicine, make sure the facilitators are well-trained and support plant sustainability and local communities. You can ask: "Where do you get your ayahuasca from?" This matters because the ayahuasca vine takes a long time to mature and has been overharvested due to the recent explosion of interest in this medicine. Do not use this medicine frivolously. It is a treasure.

HUACHUMA CACTUS: THE GRANDFATHER

The mescaline-containing huachuma or wachuma cactus, also known as San Pedro, has been used for over three thousand years in the Andes Mountains.[6] *Huachumeros* and curanderos use this sacrament in community rituals and for healing.

Many people find huachuma to be a subtle yet penetrating medicine. At lower doses, it isn't visionary, but at a certain threshold, it becomes highly visionary. You may not be able to move or talk, and you can be taken into a dreamlike visionary realm. Huachuma is excellent for introspection, group ceremony, and one-on-one therapeutic work. Many people find it especially effective for emotional release and healing the heart.

It's often dried or cooked, though occasionally eaten raw. Each type of preparation affects its ease of digestion, which matters because it can cause nausea and a bellyache. This is a medicine with a very long duration—often ten to twelve hours or longer. The experience can be intense in part because it just keeps going.

Wild huachuma cactus is endangered in northern Peru due to overharvesting and export as well as land clearing for cattle grazing.[7] Avoid contributing to this problem by sourcing only sustainably harvested San Pedro powder.

Fortunately, it can be planted and grown sustainably in supportive climates and can be found as an ornamental succulent at nurseries worldwide.

GRANDFATHER PEYOTE

The peyote cactus contains mescaline and is also addressed as "Grandfather." Peyote grows in northern Mexico and the Rio Grande Valley in the United States. It is endangered and legally protected in the United States, where it's reserved for regulated use by the Native American Church and their guests in traditional ceremonial settings.[8] The overharvesting of peyote by non-Indigenous people has threatened this sacred medicine, and the clear request from the Native American Church is to leave peyote for their use.

KETAMINE: THE DEEP RESET

Ketamine, also known as K, was first synthesized in 1962 and is considered a dissociative anesthetic, meaning it separates the mind from the body. However, it has psychedelic-like effects within a certain dosage range. While it has a long history as a recreational drug, ketamine has become popular for its antidepressant effects and ability to offer relief from anxiety and pain.[9]

The ketamine experience typically lasts about an hour, making it more accessible for some people. It can be administered in multiple ways, including as an oral lozenge, through an IV, via injection into a muscle, or as a nasal spray. Different methods produce varying intensities and onset speeds, and the resulting experiences can be quite distinct.

Because of the way it works in your brain, ketamine can help rapidly rebuild neural connections weakened by depression. Its antidepressant effects last far longer than the substance remains in your system, persisting two to four weeks or longer, as it triggers long-lasting changes in your synaptic connections. Ketamine treatment has shown a unique ability to offer both immediate and long-term relief from suicidal thoughts for those struggling with depression, something antidepressants can't do.[10]

Because it lends itself to introspection, ketamine is also offered alongside therapy, typically called ketamine-assisted psychotherapy (KAP). Many find this to be an effective approach for healing, and some practitioners combine it with gentle bodywork. At lower doses, ketamine is less likely to bring up challenging memories. Instead it can help you integrate events from the past that are already conscious. Even when painful memories do arise, many people find that ketamine's pain-relieving quality makes these memories easier to take in.

"But it's a dissociative!" people exclaim. Yes, at high doses, ketamine can create an experience of detachment from your body and environment, which is why it's used in surgery as anesthesia. However, at lower doses and when used with therapy, many people find that ketamine offers helpful distance from painful material. This is why at low doses it can be a good starting medicine for people with a trauma history: It can help you "step back" and look at fears or difficult memories without becoming overwhelmed. Many clinicians advise caution for people with a history of dissociative trauma.

Because physicians can legally prescribe ketamine, it's currently the most accessible psychedelic medicine for therapeutic use in the United States. Ketamine is being used widely in psychiatry and psychotherapy and can be combined with most psychiatric medications. As mentioned in chapter 2, it can become addictive due to its physical and emotional numbing effects.

Although ketamine-associated deaths are reported, these typically involve other substances. When people receive a proper medical screening and take ketamine with professional supervision, adverse events are rare.[11] Long-term regular use of ketamine, particularly in high doses, can cause a condition known as ketamine bladder syndrome, which is often reversible, though some cases can lead to permanent damage. However, ketamine can be fatal when combined with other substances, particularly alcohol, anxiety medications like Xanax or Valium, and opioids, or when used in an unsafe setting like a hot tub.

MDMA: HEART MEDICINE

3,4-methylenedioxymethamphetamine (MDMA), known as molly or ecstasy, is often called an entactogen or empathogen because it increases bonding hormones and the desire for closeness and connection. Its common effects include increased energy, open-heartedness, and euphoria. The experience typically lasts four to five hours. MDMA is not a "classic" psychedelic like LSD and mushrooms; technically it's an amphetamine. It rarely opens visionary or transpersonal spaces, although it can at higher doses. Your sense of self and the world don't change dramatically. Most people still feel like themselves—just their best selves.

MDMA appears to calm the amygdala (the part of your brain that processes fear and anxiety) while you remain lucid. This allows people to revisit traumatic memories and anxiety-causing situations with less fear and more objectivity. Some people call it "truth medicine" for this reason. During an MDMA experience, it's possible to think about even the most painful memories from multiple perspectives and create a new understanding around them.

MDMA has been studied extensively for its potential to reduce PTSD symptoms, and many studies describe people's dramatic shift in relationship to their traumatic memories—sometimes to the point of no longer qualifying for a PTSD diagnosis.[12] MDMA combines exceptionally well with therapy because it enhances self-reflection and insight, especially into behaviors and relationships. It's also frequently used in couples work and for working with grief.

One client described his MDMA experience as feeling like both an adult and a toddler at the same time. He "watched" memories of his parents verbally battle as they prepared to divorce. During his experience he felt clear, openhearted, and able to empathize with both his parents' pain and his frightened younger self simutaneously.

Any medication or supplement that affects serotonin can have a serious interaction with MDMA, so if you are taking any of these, you need to be evaluated prior to working with this medicine. After taking MDMA, you can feel run-down and emotional for a few days while your brain rebuilds its neurotransmitter stores. If you are healthy, you will recover within a week, so plan accordingly and give yourself a few days to rest. An intense journey can be a workout.

LSD: THE MIRROR

Lysergic acid diethylamide (LSD) is also known as acid or Lucy, while some people call it "the mirror." This medicine is considered semisynthetic because it's derived from the ergot fungus. It becomes psychoactive at the minuscule dose of 10 micrograms (0.01 mg)—about half the weight of a grain of sand![13] Yet its effects are enormous. You can feel clear-headed and present or enter visionary states. It truly is like a microscope for the mind, and if you learn to focus it, it can reveal things at the subtlest level. Albert Hofmann, the Swiss chemist who discovered LSD in 1943, described its effects this way:

> LSD simultaneously stimulates all five of our senses. You see colors more intensely, you hear better. . . . It is almost as if someone who has been blind before is suddenly able to see. After all, our consciousness is generated by everything that comes in through our sensory organs. If these sensory organs—"the doors of perception"—are opened, then you see a different world. If they then are opened too wide, you'll see hell. If you open just the right amount, you'll see heaven.[14]

LSD's effects last eight to twelve hours despite the drug leaving your bloodstream much faster. Because of the extended duration of the experience, you have the opportunity to go quite deep. There's less of a rush than shorter-acting medicines—you hang out longer with an expanded consciousness, so you have more time to work with what comes up. Of course, this also means it takes more energy to stay with what emerges.

LSD is well-suited for introspection when used in therapeutic doses, and many guides consider it ideal for exploring psychological issues. For someone who is psychologically prepared and well supported, LSD tends to have minimal side effects besides fatigue afterward. That said, LSD at higher doses can be psychologically intense, and any experience with it should be with a guide specifically trained to work with this medicine. As its nickname, "the mirror," suggests, an LSD experience tends to be open, reflective, and nonbiased. Your mind and its contents can unfold in many directions. You will need integration support after a high-dose LSD experience.

LSD was extensively studied between the 1950s and the 1970s for its ability to alleviate anxiety, depression, and addiction. When LSD became associated with 1960s counterculture and antiestablishment movements, government response was swift: The substance was criminalized in 1970, and research was effectively banned for decades. Current research with LSD is limited, though it is increasing.

5-MEO-DMT: THE DISSOLUTION

5-MeO-DMT, also known as the jaguar or the toad, exists in certain plants, as a secretion of the Sonoran Desert toad, and in a synthetic form. Because over-harvesting of the toad harms wild populations and causes animal suffering, it's recommended to use the synthetic version. Using the synthetic version also allows more precise dosing, which is critical with this medicine. While its cousin *N,N*-DMT creates vivid imagery, 5-MeO-DMT users often describe an immense spaciousness, tremendous power, and a purifying quality. It can be heart-opening and loving or frightening and overwhelming. It's not uncommon to feel oneself dissolving or having an out-of-body experience. Current research is looking at 5-MeO-DMT's potential for anxiety and depression.

This medicine is one of the most intense and rapidly acting psychedelic substances available. The experience is brief, often just fifteen to twenty minutes, though those minutes can feel like an eternity. Because the experience happens so quickly, there's usually no sense of relating to other people during the journey. You can be launched into an entirely different dimension of consciousness.

5-MeO-DMT's cousin bufotenin (5-HO-DMT) exists naturally, along with a small amount of 5-MeO-DMT, in psychoactive seeds in South America. These seeds, known as *yopo*, *cohoba*, *cebil*, or *vilca*, are typically used as snuff and have been used for healing and prayer for over four thousand years.[15]

These are not medicines for beginners. I do not recommend you work with these medicines unless you are experienced with other psychedelics, are being guided by someone well-trained, and are prepared for their intensity. Supportive integration afterward is essential.

WHAT I HAVEN'T COVERED

The medicines I've focused on are the most researched and widely available in contemporary psychedelic healing. Many other plant medicines and synthetic compounds exist—some with thousands of years of traditional use, others developed in recent decades. Each has its own character, risks, and healing potential, but I haven't covered them because they're either less accessible, require more specialized knowledge, or have less research establishing their safety and efficacy. If you're drawn to explore beyond the medicines described earlier, do thorough research and seek guidance from experienced practitioners.

Ibogaine deserves special mention. Derived from the iboga plant used in Bwiti ceremonies in Central Africa, ibogaine has shown remarkable potential for treating opioid addiction—sometimes able to help people reset their relationship with opioids in a single session.[16] However, it carries serious cardiovascular risks and requires careful medical screening and monitoring. If you're considering ibogaine for addiction recovery, work only with experienced professionals who can assess your heart health and provide proper supervision.

Which Medicine Calls You?

Each psychedelic medicine is a unique sacrament that brings its own gifts. As with people, you may find some more harmonious with your constitution than others. You are entering into a relationship that builds over time. Just because you have one experience does not mean you know that medicine. It just means you have met. Keep showing up if you want to go deeper.

A few questions to consider when deciding which medicine to explore:

- Do you want to explore your life story or connect with something larger?
- Are you seeking healing, exploration, or spiritual connection?
- Do you prefer gradual revelation or sudden breakthrough?
- Do you need your thinking mind to stay somewhat online, or are you ready for dissolution?
- How much emotional upheaval can you handle right now?
- Are you in a stable enough place to have your worldview shifted?
- Do you have space in your life for several days or weeks of integration?

Your choice of medicine, along with where, how, and with whom you work, will directly shape your experience.

After you've decided on a setting and identified which medicine calls to you, it's time to enter the active phase of preparation. If you're attending a ceremony, working with a trained guide, or heading to a legal psilocybin center, the facilitator should help you prepare. If you're journeying on your own, you'll need to create this structure yourself. In the next chapter, I'll walk you through ways to prepare your body, mind, and heart for a psychedelic journey.

CHAPTER 6
Preparing for Your Journey

Tania was in her mid-forties and arrived at my office in a sleeveless floral blouse, slacks, and heels. Her short bob, pearl earrings, and red lips completed her polished look. She seemed quite nervous. "How can I help you?" I asked after we exchanged introductions.

She sat up straighter and glanced around the room. "Well, I took mushrooms twice recently, and they absolutely cracked me open."

"Oh, was this with a guide or friends or . . ."

"Oh, no! I got them from a friend, but I took them alone . . . at home . . . while my husband was at work and the kids were at school."

My eyes widened. "How old are your kids?"

"Five-year-old twins and an eight-year-old."

"How was it? And how much did you take?"

"To tell you the truth, it was terrible. I took a little the first time. That was okay. Then a week later I finished the bag. I don't know how much it was, but I got super scared and thought I was dying. I thought about calling for help but talked myself out of it. All I could think about was how everything is going to end. I'm going to die, my kids are going to die, and everything . . ." She leaned in and lowered her voice to a whisper. "Everything and everyone . . . is going to die." She blinked at me with tears in her eyes as we sat together quietly for a few moments.

"That's a big journey." I nudged the tissue box closer to her. "Was this your first experience?"

She nodded. "I was a straight-A student through college, a perfect daughter, then the perfect wife and mom for the last nine years. For years, my life has been grocery shopping, laundry, and bedtime stories. A year ago, I started feeling trapped. I watched a documentary about psychedelic mushrooms and couldn't stop thinking about them. It was like they were calling me. A friend mentioned he could get me some, and I went for it."

I nodded. I could certainly understand why she would seek this out.

"It was intense. I think I took too much. It was all about death and how everything will die, and there's nothing I can do about it. Now, I keep thinking about losing my kids, and I just feel so tense." She looked down and continued: "I just keep wondering what the point of it all is, if it's all going to end. I'm not suicidal or anything—I want to be alive. I just don't see the point if we all die alone in the end."

I listened, appreciating her sincerity. "So you jumped right in, and it doesn't sound like you had much time to prepare."

"Prepare? Well, I watched that documentary. I talked to my friend about his journeys. He's had quite a few. And then I waited for a day when my husband was at work and the kids had after-school care. But besides that, no."

"It's good you didn't do it while your kids were home!"

She laughed.

"Did you have an intention for your experience?"

"Not really. I've been curious and feeling lost, but nothing beyond that. I know it was impulsive." She looked at me with a bit of guilt. "I'm a private person, and it just seemed like the easiest way to do it—by myself at home."

I shook my head. "No judgment at all. I'm impressed. You didn't know what you were getting into. I'm glad you're here now."

She shook her head. "I had no idea."

Tania and I worked together for three months. She eventually shared that her beloved grandmother had died suddenly two years earlier, a loss she hadn't fully grieved. As we talked, she began to see how her journey had brought her grief to the surface. I helped her design a healing ritual where she wrote a letter to her grandmother and buried it at the beach with her family. Eventually, she felt she had come through her experience. She decided to work with a guide for her next journey.

Tania isn't alone in diving headfirst into an experience with sacred medicine without guidance or preparation. She was in good psychological health, so the material she encountered, although painful, didn't seriously destabilize her. She was struggling afterward, but as soon as she had a place to talk, things smoothed out.

I live at the base of Mt. Shasta, a 14,000-foot snow-capped mountain that attracts adventurers and spiritual pilgrims year-round. Occasionally we hear of people attempting to summit unprepared, arriving in running shoes with a few snacks, claiming they were "called to the mountain." Some of these attempts, as you might imagine, end badly. Similarly, a psychedelic journey is a considerable endeavor that requires preparation. The last few chapters have described various routes up the mountain. Now, before you embark, you should check the conditions and have the right gear. Wise climbers know that even if they are diligent and careful, accidents can still happen. But if things line up, they can look forward to a strenuous yet ultimately rewarding climb to the summit.

Preparation makes a real difference. Let's explore how you can best prepare both practically and internally for your journey.

Why Prepare?

The way we prepare for a journey strongly influences its outcome. Most of us live rushing from one demand to another: work, grocery shopping, kids, dogs, house, and car repairs. Even those who live in the country have their hands full planting the garden, fixing the well, and tending animals. Slowing down long enough to prepare for a psychedelic journey is an act of pushing back against this rushing river of demands. It takes determination to carve out time, reflect on what lies ahead, and craft an intention, but your effort will be rewarded.

If you're working with a guide, they'll likely walk you through your preparation. If you're planning a self-guided journey, it's up to you. Many traditional cultures include preparation practices before ceremonies: cleansing, fasting, or isolation.[1] Current research confirms that time spent on preparation, especially building the relationship between facilitators and participants, correlates with therapeutic outcomes.[2] In over fifteen years of guiding journeys, I've witnessed this difference firsthand.

Preparation includes ensuring you're medically safe to proceed and as physically, emotionally, mentally, and spiritually ready as possible. The goal isn't to guarantee an effortless or mystical experience; that isn't possible. However, you can set yourself up to engage sincerely and wholeheartedly with whatever arises. There are three major benefits:

Safety and risk reduction: Many, though not all, adverse experiences can be avoided or minimized with better preparation. If you are working with a guide, their job is to track early signs that you aren't physically or psychologically ready. When you prepare carefully, red flags can emerge and receive the attention they need. Sometimes the right decision is to slow down, take extra time, or postpone the journey.

Respect for the medicine: When you interact with a power that can help or harm you, showing your sincerity is wise. Taking time to prepare honors the people who grew, harvested, or synthesized the medicine, and if you're working with a guide, respects their efforts on your behalf. This makes for a more sustainable relationship with the medicine.

Showing up settled and clear: When you take time to catch up with yourself and digest recent events—the argument with your partner, the news story weighing on you, the project you just completed—you clear space inside. If your inner world is crowded with unintegrated experiences, those will likely surface during your journey. Ask yourself: What's really up for me now? What am I actually ready to look at?

The Three Phases of Preparation

Following are the three phases you will move through in your preparation.

LAYING THE GROUNDWORK

Self-Assessment and Research

Long-term preparation begins when you first consider seeking a psychedelic experience. You're reading this book, watching online videos, asking friends about their journeys, and contemplating whether this type of healing would be good for you. This is a good time to take my self-assessment questionnaire (see appendix A) and see if you're ready. If you are medically safe and ready to proceed, educate yourself about options: Read this book and others, and learn what's available in your area. Ask questions like: When do I want to have an experience, and where? What medicine do I hope to work with? Do I want to work with a guide?

Medical and Safety Planning

Even if you've been medically and psychologically cleared to move forward, if you have health concerns or a sensitive mental health history, think through how a journey might affect you. If you have an autoimmune condition, you might have a flare-up after your journey. If you sink into a depressive episode, what kind of support will you want in place? If you plan to revisit a traumatic event or past abuse, set up extra layers of care for the two weeks after your journey. You may feel quite raw and need emotional support. An experienced guide should help you think through these concerns, but it's also good to plan to take care of yourself in case they miss something.

Build Capacity and Find Your Anchors

Preparation for a high-dose session should include cultivating your ability to stay present with intense sensations and emotions in your body and mind. During your journey, you might reach the limits of your usual control. How can you intentionally develop your capacity to stay open in these moments? What practices will help you return to your center?

Consider finding an introductory meditation class or a weekend breath-work workshop, or spending ten minutes each day practicing belly breathing, a simple technique that can help you stabilize quickly. Develop a visualization or image that speaks to you: yourself as a tree with deep roots extending into the earth, or a bird you love soaring through the sky. Look for a prayer or mantra that connects you to something larger than yourself. Think of friends or family members who are always there for you. Establishing these anchors beforehand will give you a lifeline when things get turbulent.

You can also start thinking about your intention. It's never too early to get in touch with your deeper reasons for seeking a psychedelic journey.

TWO WEEKS OUT

Short-term preparation begins when you have a journey on your schedule and at least two weeks to prepare. Consider spending an hour preparing for every hour you will spend in your journey. For example, if you are getting ready for a mushroom journey, which typically lasts around five hours, see if you can dedicate the same amount of time to preparing. These hours can include reading or watching documentaries about psychedelics and plant medicine, engaging in preparation sessions with your guide, spending quiet time in a natural setting you love, journaling, or using your art supplies for creative visioning. Ask yourself: What do I need to do to arrive at my journey prepared logistically, physically, and emotionally? As much as you can, give your preparation focused attention.

Building Rapport with Your Guide

If you're working with a guide, they should be actively building rapport with you as you move toward your scheduled date through in-person meetings, phone calls, or emails. If you don't have enough time scheduled to get to know one another before your session, request more time. Cultivating a sense of trust with your guide will help you relax and be more comfortable turning inward.

Plan for Spaciousness

What can you do in advance to ensure a spacious week leading up to your journey? If you can, schedule the day before off from work and responsibilities, and ideally one to two days afterward. That means no appointments or firm commitments. This way you can still choose to have lunch with a friend or go for a hike, but you aren't obligated to do so. You may find yourself just wanting to rest, stare into space, or write in your journal. If you can't afford time off but want alone time to integrate before returning to a busy home, can you spend one night at a hotel or a friend's house?

THE FINAL WEEK

Immediate preparation is when your journey is scheduled within the coming week.

Let Your Mind and Body Settle

Letting your body and mind settle and move into a receptive state before a journey will help you be available for what is coming. Consider refraining from overstimulating activities, difficult-to-digest foods, alcohol, psychoactive substances, distressing media, exhausting people, and anything else that destabilizes you. If scrolling through social media or reading the news makes you furious, take a week-long break before your journey. If dinner with your in-laws leaves you frustrated, skip it this week. They'll be fine.

Rest is also essential. When we give it permission, our body naturally gravitates toward what it needs. If you arrive at your journey exhausted, you might find yourself sinking into a trance-like slumber. If you want an experience that is more dynamic than a few hours of restorative sleep, make sure you show up with plenty of energy. If you are feeling sick, reschedule.

Preparing for Your Return

On a practical level, plan for a low-stress return and consider ways to make your home as comfortable as possible. You will likely feel more emotional and open after your journey, and you'll want to savor that feeling. Let any housemates or family members know that you will need extra space: no bad news, no demands, no heavy conversations for a day or two. Finish anything awaiting completion beforehand and tie up loose ends so you won't be pulled back into work or chores.

What food do you want in the fridge when you get back? You will likely fast from food until evening on your journey day, and your senses will be awake in a way you can only imagine. The coconut water and tomato soup you prepared ahead might be the most delicious meal you've ever had.

Protection and Intention

You want to be protective of yourself following your journey, as extended suggestibility can make you especially sensitive to external influences. If you make plans for later in the week, limit them to friends, family, and activities that are inspiring and relaxing, not demanding. Consider telling people now that you may want to connect with them afterward; it's great to have people on call, ready to support you if needed.

Start thinking about protective forces you can call on during your journey. These can include mentors, ancestors, spiritual deities, animals, or elements of nature. They might be your great-grandmother, a mountain you love, a white tiger, or the goddess Kali. Who or what gives you strength and a sense of being fiercely protected?

This is also the time to connect with your motivation and get precise with your intention, which I talk about in the next chapter.

The Days Before

In the days leading up to your journey, focus on activities that help you feel grounded and steady: Take a walk, do some stretching, or enjoy a morning of meditation or coffee and journaling. Pay attention to your dreams and track any unusual signs or synchronicities. Note any animals you see, unexpected interactions you have, and anything else that catches your eye. You can share your notes with your guide or contemplate their meaning on your own.

As for preparing your body, fasting before a plant-medicine ceremony has been practiced in traditional settings for centuries. Many people find that fasting reduces nausea and enhances the effects of the medicine. Arrive with an empty stomach unless your guide tells you otherwise. If you have low blood sugar, consider having a small, easily digested meal such as toast, yogurt, or a banana early in the morning. Wear comfortable clothing with nothing tight or restrictive. Make sure you have a bottle of water and plenty of warm layers.

If you are restless and don't sleep well the night before, don't worry. This is common, and it usually won't affect your journey. On the day of your journey, it's normal to feel nervous. If you can, imagine the best possible outcomes. Reaffirm your intention and trust your deeper motivation, letting the truth of that support you.

Setting-Specific Preparation

GROUP CEREMONY

Some group ceremony facilitators include extensive preparation, while others provide very little. Some are happy to have a phone call, while others may want to meet in person before you join their group. Others run large groups frequently and don't make themselves available to connect beforehand. They might only ask you to read their guidelines or be accompanied by a seasoned participant who will orient you.

Meeting the facilitators and assistants, understanding everyone's roles, and reviewing group agreements and ceremony rules will help you relax, so try to do so if you can. Ask about the basic schedule so you know what to expect. Some ceremonies start at 6 p.m. and run exactly five hours, while others begin at 11 p.m. and go all night, through sunrise, until everyone is complete. You want to know what you are committing to. Always be prepared for changes.

SELF-GUIDED JOURNEY

I only recommend a self-guided journey if you have considerable experience (ten or more high-dose journeys). Even then, stay in a low-dose range. In a self-guided journey, you will be playing two roles, journeyer and guide, and you should feel comfortable holding both. You're taking on more complexity and must handle all the responsibilities typically managed by a facilitator while also being in an expanded state of consciousness.

Ensure you've researched risks and contraindications, obtained clean medicine with known potency, created a safe and comfortable environment, and have one to two friends you can call for support.

Consider looking for an online or local psychedelic integration circle ahead of time for post-journey support. You can call a psychedelic support hotline if you need immediate help during your journey. For true medical emergencies, call 911.

Open or Closed Eyes: Do You Really Need an Eye Mask?

Some guides are very strict about using eye masks. However, I believe you should always have the choice of whether to close your eyes or keep them open. People have been journeying without eye masks for thousands of years; it is entirely possible to have a full experience with your eyes open, closed, or moving between the two. Do what feels right for you.

What are the benefits of wearing an eye mask? Blocking out visual distraction can direct your attention inward. Can you just put an old scarf over your eyes? Of course. But if you're someone who gets easily distracted by even small amounts of light, an eye mask can help. It may intensify your experience, but it can also help you go deeper and move through whatever is happening. Otherwise, you can get stuck at the surface and spin in circles. Recent research also suggests that closing your eyes during a psychedelic journey may enhance the experience.[3]

However, certain encounters only happen if your eyes are open. During an outdoor mushroom journey, I once had a hummingbird come and hover right in front of my face for what seemed like minutes, the two of us staring into each other's eyes. I could feel her high-frequency vibration penetrating my forehead. I can't remember much else about that day, but the moment with the hummingbird stays with me years later.

The Limits of Preparation

The nature of any initiatory experience is to encounter the unknown. It spontaneously calls forth inner resources and capacities you didn't know you had. Even if you do your best to prepare for a voyage into the unknown, ultimately, it's unpredictable. That's part of the point and the magic.

A psychedelic journey is like a divination. The outcome responds to countless variables: your mood, biochemical reactions, the weather outside, and the songs you hear. It's impossible to know in advance how these factors will interact and where they will take you. The tension between preparation and willing surrender is central to this work. You can take steps to be as ready as possible, but hold it lightly; preparation has its limits. And yet, a certain grace always seems to appear for those who come with humility and sincerity.

Are You Prepared?

- What is your motivation for seeking a psychedelic experience at this time?
- Do you know the effects and potential aftereffects of the substance that will be your sacrament for the day?
- Do you know whom you will be with, and do you trust them to provide support if you need it?
- Do you know where you will be, and do you feel confident that you will be safe and relaxed there?
- Do you have safe transportation set up?
- Do you have everything you might need? At a minimum, bring warm layers, water, snacks, a headlamp, and a phone to stay in touch if needed.
- Do you have a comfortable place to return to afterward?

- Do you have integration support set up? A facilitator or therapist to check in with, a day to rest and reflect, or friends to reach out to?
- Is this the right moment? If you have any doubts, pause and check in with yourself before crossing the threshold. Considering the intensity of a psychedelic journey, I encourage you to give credence to any hesitation you feel.

What do you need to do to arrive at your journey relaxed, alert, and receptive, with as much self-awareness as possible? Healing work can be tumultuous; the psyche can be a dark, stormy sea. You may encounter weather. Arriving prepared, you can raise your sail high into the wind, your prayer written upon the waving canvas. Even if you don't know your final destination, your compass will guide you, helping you stay centered despite the strong wind. Your direction may need to change mid-voyage—not a problem. Adjust your sails, bow to the open ocean, and steer with the wind. An adventure awaits.

CHAPTER 7
Crafting Your Intention

The most important thing is to find out what is the most important thing.

—SUZUKI ROSHI

Marcela took a long pull on her hand-rolled tobacco cigar and lifted her head, blowing smoke toward the sky. She was sitting across from me on a white plastic chair in her family compound deep in the Peruvian rainforest, her feet planted on the dusty earth below. She cracked the lightest of smiles, revealing a glimpse of her gold teeth. She looked right at me and asked, *"¿Y qué pediste? ¿Cuál fue tu rezo?"* (Well, what did you ask for? What was your prayer?)

What *had* I asked for? What had I whispered into the cup of ayahuasca, the thick brown brew I held in my hands before blowing tobacco smoke on it and swallowing it down? It was just last night, yet it felt light-years away. Closing my eyes catapulted me back into visions still fresh from the night's ceremony. I had been in a world of birds. Feathered creatures of every color flew in circles above me as I sat still in the center of a grove of luminous trees. They trilled a thousand melodies at once, creating a cacophony of song. I tried to move, but felt glued to the earth below me. I tried to make a sound, but nothing came. Suddenly everything stopped, birds hovering in perfect stillness. Gray squirrels, red foxes, shimmering blue butterflies—creatures emerged from every direction, and a feeling of immense love enveloped me. It was magnificent—but what had been my prayer? What did I ask for?

I hadn't asked for anything. I had flown 4,500 miles to Lima, then traveled another 500 miles by bus, followed by a four-hour boat ride to this small village in the Amazon because I was curious and seeking something, though I wasn't sure what. Now I felt embarrassed. I told her the truth: I hadn't asked for anything. Marcela squinted at me with amusement in her eyes, then gazed off into the distance, laughed softly, and shook her head. *"Está bien."* (It's fine.)

In retrospect, I wish I had taken the time to reflect more carefully on my motivation so I could connect what I had seen to an inquiry. All I could say was that it was spectacular, but not connected to anything I could articulate.

If you are fortunate enough to find your way to a ceremony or journey with a potent medicine, in a safe place with a seasoned guide or even by yourself, you have a precious opportunity. Ask yourself: What do I want to look at more deeply? What do I want to let go of? What am I calling into my life?

An intention is not about what you want "out there." An intention isn't about fixing external circumstances or controlling outcomes. It's about clarifying what you want to understand, embody, or shift within yourself. Getting clear on this means taking time to reflect on your day-to-day life and deciding where to cast your focus before entering an expanded state of consciousness.

As you prepare for a psychedelic journey, your intention can serve as an arrow guiding your way forward, helping you clarify your next steps. If you are working with a guide, it can help them understand your goals so they can focus their support. During your journey, your intention can be a touchstone you return to if everything else falls away. The words of your intention may fall away as well—no need to grasp them; you can return to them afterward. You can also ask your guide to remind you of your intention during your experience. During integration, recalling your intention can help enrich your understanding of why specific images, messages, or insights came to you.

You can approach your intention as an inquiry question, an aspirational prayer, or a wish. Taking the time to craft your intention acknowledges that you are in communication with something larger than yourself, whether that's your own unconscious mind, the greater natural world, the sentient spirit of the medicine, the greater field of Love, or the Great Mystery.

Why Use an Intention?

Crafting a deliberate intention brings you to the center of your journey, balancing the tendency to over-rely on a guide, the medicine, or the outcome. It's easy to over-focus on a destination and forget that your motivation shapes how your journey unfolds. An intention keeps the focus on the greater arc you are traveling, regardless of what happens in any given moment.

As mentioned in chapter 1, psychedelics increase neuroplasticity—the brain's capacity to form new neural connections and pathways. Forming an intention before your journey seeds your subconscious with a specific direction, guiding your attention. While suggestibility has a shadow, you can use self-suggestion for good. An intention can harness what's sometimes called the placebo effect—the well-documented phenomenon in which believing in something strongly contributes to a positive outcome.[1] When you bring your clear intention into a neuroplastic state, you're creating conditions that can support real change. An intention you've consciously crafted will resonate through all the layers of your being, helping you align with your direction. Recalling your intention in a critical moment can cut through any trance of distraction or self-delusion, giving you the capacity to respond rather than react.

People with a more scientific view may wonder if they even need an intention. They ask: "If clinical trials have proven that psilocybin relieves depression, and that's what I'm coming for, why do I need to ask for anything?" From a strictly materialist viewpoint, the medicine should work regardless. Yet expectation significantly influences outcome—a well-established effect.

Others ask: "Can't I just see what happens? I'd rather leave it to the mystery." Like I did that night in Peru, many seekers set off on pilgrimage out of curiosity, without knowing exactly what they're after. Forgoing an intention is fine if that feels right, and arriving without one won't hurt you. But even an intention as simple as "Please teach me" or "I want to explore" can guide your trajectory.

Taking time to craft an intention is an offering to the medicine and to your own deeper being. It shows you are sincere, as it requires humility to admit you need help. It shows both yourself and "the powers that be" that you are willing to give your time, money, and comfort to ask beyond yourself for help, knowing you may not get a response, or that the response may not be what you hope for. So what in your life do you want to illuminate?

Three Types of Intention

There are as many types of intentions as there are people seeking journeys. When crafting yours, consider these three areas of focus: healing, vision, or gratitude.

A HEALING INTENTION

Many people come to psychedelic journeys seeking relief from depression, anxiety, chronic migraines, insomnia, or addiction. If your intention is physical healing, you can ask for it: "Please show me the direction of my healing," or even just "Heal me." Or you could ask an inquiry question like: "What do I need to do or understand to strengthen my physical vitality and health?" You may gain insight into how habits, stressful relationships, or social pressures are contributing to your health problems.

Sometimes you are given a larger view and can see how the forces at play are impacting you. Losing your job, surviving childhood abuse, or being the target of discrimination are factors that are out of your control. Here, your intention might evolve: "How can I respond to my situation in a way that doesn't make me ill?" or "What support do I need to navigate this with less stress?"

To be fair, psychedelic journeys are not a surefire miracle cure for physical healing. Fixating on getting rid of physical symptoms can become an obstacle. I did integration sessions with Claire, a woman in her fifties with early-stage multiple sclerosis. She wanted support as she joined a local group for a series of three mushroom ceremonies, each a month apart, to see if it would help her symptoms. She was tired after the first two and decided that was enough. She told me, "I realized in both journeys that it's not about getting rid of my symptoms; it's about learning to live with this condition more gracefully. It's not going away. I don't like it, but I need to learn how to let this be my teacher." Sometimes there is dramatic physical healing, and other times there is no shift in your physical condition. Either way, the experience can still be life-changing.

AN INTENTION TO SEEK VISION

Even when life is swimming along—healthy relationships, steady purpose and work, or even leisure—there's usually something new to discover or further refine. In this case, you can seek guidance or a vision for the next step in your life. Your intention might be: "What comes next?"

My friend Mohan was in his early forties, working in event production, and eager to have an LSD journey before his wife gave birth to their second child. I encouraged him to seek a guide, which he did, and then helped him craft his intention. He explained how stressful it had been to be a first-time parent, with many fights with his wife over how much he was working. His intention was simple: "Please show me how to be as prepared as I can be for our new baby—what do I need to see, learn, or do to be the best husband and father I can be?"

Mohan said he had a vision of all the nights he had stayed late at work, constantly pushing himself to get ahead in his career. He realized his obsession with success was actually an attempt to be validated by his own father, who was emotionally distant. He said he saw how clueless he was about how to be a good father, and that his career was where he felt confident. He told me he got a direct answer to his intention: "Stop trying to impress your father; it's never going to happen. Give yourself to your family and trust that you'll figure it out."

He realized he didn't need to be perfect. He just needed to be humble.

Who did you come here to be, and what did you come here to do? In what new way might you grow further into your potential as a human being, or as part of the greater web of being?

AN INTENTION OF GRATITUDE

Many people don't realize they can show up for a journey with an intention of gratitude. They think they need a problem. It's true that conditions of ease rarely shape our lives, and it's easier to focus on what's lacking. However, the exquisite intention of offering appreciation is about giving thanks for what you have. This may be appropriate when you're in a season of abundant health or wealth, or after an accomplishment.

Robin was a client who wanted help preparing for an ayahuasca ceremony she had been invited to. She had just completed a drawn-out divorce and was exhausted but ready to celebrate. Robin stated her intention as: "I offer gratitude for the inner strength I tapped into, for the people who helped me, and for this new chapter of peace." During her ceremony, she had visions of the faces of the lawyers who supported her, of dark times when she somehow found the energy to keep going, and of moments of grace when friends and family had helped her. Robin told me she spent hours between gratitude and grief, with tears rolling down her face; it was just the profound release her weary body and spirit had needed.

An intention of gratitude or appreciation can be especially healing for people who struggle with self-criticism, pessimism, or cynicism, or who have a habit of believing they need to work harder, be better, or do more.

When you arrive at a journey with a full heart, not asking for anything from outside yourself, you can attract unforeseen insights or visions. Whether it's expressing appreciation for your current circumstances, celebrating a personal accomplishment, or simply thanking the medicine itself, gratitude can be a complete intention in itself.

How to Craft Your Intention

Taking the time to clarify your intention a week or so before your journey will give you time to refine it. Start by setting aside one to two hours. Silence external distractions or go somewhere you can be alone to reflect on your life and contemplate why you are seeking a journey. Many people find writing helpful for connecting with subconscious longings and bringing them to the surface. If you're not the journaling type, work with color and images in a notebook with unlined paper.

Breathe into your belly and let yourself settle. Close your eyes and listen inward. Reflect on your life, including close relationships, work stressors, and issues you are struggling with. Beyond the problems you want solutions for, scan your life for areas that feel dull or neglected. Maybe it's your relationship with a sibling, your neglected writing project, or a feeling that you're treading water and have no larger vision that lights you up. Also reflect on parts of your life that make you smile and fill your heart—your kids, your dogs, drinking green tea in the morning, or your favorite spot in the wilderness.

As you settle into a reflective space, contemplate these questions:

HEALING

- Do you want to look more closely into recurring conflicts with a partner, friend, child, or parent?
- Are you healing from a recent breakup?
- Is there a physical health issue or persistent mood you want to explore?
- Are you grieving a deceased parent, spouse, friend, or pet?
- Are you looking to heal ancestral trauma?
- Are you processing childhood abuse or neglect, or a traumatic event from your past?
- Is the state of the world impacting your well-being?

VISION

- Are you preparing for a move, career change, or retirement and hoping to understand what the next phase of your life might bring?
- Are you preparing to get married or to become a parent?
- Are you seeking a romantic relationship?

- Are you seeking artistic inspiration or wrestling with creative blocks?
- Are you looking for ways to be of service or to become more politically active?
- Do you need guidance on your role in a relationship that is struggling?

GRATITUDE

- Is there anything you've recently accomplished or completed that you want to celebrate?
- Have you received support or guidance that deserves your acknowledgment?
- Do you want to appreciate something you might be taking for granted in a specific relationship, community, or with yourself?

If these questions don't quite land, try free-writing with one of the following prompts. Write the beginning of the sentence and then let yourself complete it. Try writing it out fifteen times to see if your answers deepen as you progress.

- I'm ready to let go of . . .
- What I crave most in my life right now is . . .
- The areas of my life that need more attention or vitality are . . .
- I want to shed more light on . . .
- What feels most in tension in my life right now is . . .
- What is pulling at the strings of my heart right now is . . .
- The images and feelings coming to me in my waking and sleeping dreams are . . .

Review what you wrote and try to uncover the main theme, the core, the pith of it all.

Once you have a sense of your focus, summarize your intention in one to three sentences that express an inquiry or a prayer of aspiration. For example:

- **Inquiry**: "What silences my voice in relationships, and how can I find the courage to speak my truth with honesty and love?"

- **Aspiration**: "May I see what silences my voice in relationships and find my courage so I can begin to speak from honesty and love."

Distill the words down to their essence and tweak each sentence until your intention resonates with brilliant clarity and makes you exclaim, "Yes!" in a way you can feel.

Make sure to create an intention that is fully yours. The voices in our lives—parents, older siblings, teachers, and the desires of others—have a way of burrowing into our consciousness and obscuring our true intentions. Only you know where you are on your path and what comes next. Also avoid creating an intention that has an agenda for anyone else's life. "How can I get my ex to take me back?" puts the focus on your ex. How can you change the words to be entirely focused on yourself and your role?

Watch out for intentions that are too vague or general, or that try to jam in every issue in your life. For example: "I wish to heal my relationship with my mother-in-law, call in my soulmate, decide whether to move to Austin, see what's going on with the pain in my lower back, and connect with the spirit of my dead cat, Kiwi Bear, and apologize for not taking him to the vet sooner."

Choose one focus and let the rest fall into place. Although many topics can be visited during a journey, a clear focus keeps you grounded. Remember: You are forming one intention for one journey, and there will be future opportunities. An intention shouldn't sound like a demand, but like a confident request made with humility. If it sounds like a demand, keep working on it.

A strong intention contains both active and receptive aspects. It is engaged yet open, courageous yet humble. Here are examples of intentions my clients have brought to their journeys.

- "I am deeply grateful for my wife's recovery from her stroke. I want to celebrate her renewed health and the time we have together, and integrate the last six months of being her caregiver as we step into the next phase of life together."
- "Please grant me insight into what is blocking my creativity and help me understand the fear that keeps me from returning to my painting. I'm ready to reconnect with the joy and playfulness that once fueled my creative process and step back into my artistic self."

- "What are the underlying forces keeping me and my partner stuck in conflict? I want to understand my role in our arguments and see how I can respond with love instead of reactivity."
- "I'm ready to look at my drinking. Show me what I need to get sober and what kind of support I need."
- "After months of being in a thick fog, I'm ready to see my next steps. Please grant me a vision of what to do next and how to do it. And may I have the courage to trust what I see."

If you are afraid, ask for courage. If you are unsure, ask for confidence. If you don't know what you want, ask for clarity. If you can't see the next step, ask for guidance. If it will be your first experience with a specific medicine, you can always bring a sweet, simple intention to meet it as you would a new friend. "It's good to meet you. Please introduce yourself to me and teach me about yourself."

After taking the time to craft your intention, if you still don't know what it is, that's fine. You might just need more time. Working with a guide or someone who specializes in psychedelic integration can help.

Your Intention in Action

Write your intention on a piece of paper you can touch and hold. If you aren't a word person, or if you want to add a visual element, translate your intention into a collage of images, colors, and symbols to activate your subconscious mind. You are birthing your intention from thought into form, from your heart into the material plane.

Place your written or visual intention somewhere you can see it: on your bedside table, taped to your bathroom mirror, or on a shrine or altar. If you don't have a shrine or altar, create one. An outer altar serves as a sacred portal, reflecting the inner altar of your heart. It can be elaborate or simple, featuring a few objects that hold meaning for you: a beautiful cloth, wildflowers in a small glass, a few stones, or a holy image.

For a few days before your journey, take a moment to reflect on your intention in the morning and again in the evening. Whisper it, speak it, or sing it out loud—feel it inside. If the words need to shift, change them. If you're working with a guide, share your intention with them during your final preparation meeting. Share it with others only if it feels right—keeping it private can increase its power.

Then, bring your written or drawn intention with you to your journey or ceremony. Place it on the altar or keep it folded in your pocket. Speak it out loud or quietly in your mind right before you take your medicine.

Traditional healers in the Amazon taught me to draw tobacco smoke from a hand-rolled cigarette and blow my prayer into the medicine before drinking it. You don't need tobacco; you can use your breath. Blow your intention into your medicine, ask for what you want, and call on the healing force of the medicine to activate.

One ayahuasca healer told me, "You want to ask the medicine for what you need, like you ask your neighbor for some sugar. Be polite." The plants and molecules might not hear your request the way your neighbor would, but consider the possibility that in some mysterious way, they still hear you.

Sometimes what happens in a journey doesn't seem to respond to your intention in any way. No need to be frustrated or disappointed. Magic works in mysterious ways. Sometimes no answer is the answer you need. And over time, you may begin to understand how your intention was met after all.

Bringing an intention to your journey is a way to actively engage with the interdependence of life. It's an act of taking time to pause, listen, and articulate what your soul is reaching toward or what your future self is whispering back to you.

Your intention extends beyond words on a notecard. It's your prayer, a declaration of what is alive in your heart and what matters to you at this moment in your life. Remember that developing your intention is an art, not a science. Don't become fixated on crafting the perfect intention. Just find what feels true to you right now.

As you move toward your journey or ceremony, the invitation is to hold your intention both lightly and sincerely, in a way that helps you feel anchored while remaining receptive to wherever you need to go. The medicine can respond to you in ways you never imagined, and remaining open to surprise can lead to unexpected blessings.

Trust that by naming what you're seeking, you have aligned with your deepest wish. Your intention, bright and true, will guide your way forward, not only as a reverent supplicant but also as a conscious agent in your own unfolding.

CHAPTER 8

Navigating Your Psychedelic Journey

I sit quietly on the wooden floor of the cabin. Sunlight streams in through the branches of a pine tree just outside the window. I invoke the steady power of the snow-covered mountain to my north, call in my protectors and teachers, then whisper my intention and a prayer of gratitude into the earthen mug in my hands. Taking a breath, I drink its contents—ground mushrooms blended with liquid chocolate. After twenty minutes, a wave of warmth rolls through me. I feel a gentle loosening, like a marionette whose handler has stepped away. I need to lie down.

My guide nods toward the futon. I crawl over, climb under the blanket, and reach for the eye mask. Inhaling deeply, I bring my hands to my belly.

The music begins—deep, soulful cello—and I marvel as the invisible glue holding me together begins to melt. Space seeps into my seams. A swell of emotion rises in my chest. Sorrow? Grief? It feels familiar yet foreign at the same time. Is it mine? I can't tell. It presses on me until I feel myself crack a little more. My heartbeat increases, and tears trickle from the corners of my eyes.

My grief is here now, flowing out of me, as my animal body lets down its guard. I hear birdsong and the distant roar of an airplane. I remember my intention as I exhale and let go.

⁂

A psychedelic journey can take you in countless directions. You may encounter the perplexing, the awe-inspiring, or the sublime. You may also encounter painful feelings or frightening and disturbing images. Rarely is this experience predictable or comfortable, and for this reason, it's normal to feel anxious or tentative. Like approaching the ocean's edge, you're stepping into a vast and unpredictable realm. Geometric lights, familiar faces, ancient memories, tears of rage, the wails of buried grief, unfamiliar beings, prophetic visions, waves of blissful joy, or the ecstasy of union—all are possible. How do you navigate this territory if it's new to you?

Remember that humans have been ingesting psychedelic plants for thousands of years. A long line of explorers has come before you; deep in your bones, you too can find the strength to endure the demanding parts of your journey. Your own ancestors traveled to faraway lands and crossed thresholds, not knowing what lay on the other side. Call on them to be with you now.

This chapter explores the arc of a psychedelic journey, including the five phases many journeyers move through: the ascent, the depths, the revelations and healings, the mystical dimension, and the return. I offer a kaleidoscopic view of these realms and ways to move through them.

The arc I describe here most closely reflects a psilocybin mushroom or LSD journey. The setting you are in for your journey has a great deal to do with how fully you can give yourself to your experience. If you are in a group ceremony, there may be rules around movement or making noise that require you to contain yourself more than in other settings. My suggestions align with the experience of being in a safe place with a guide or a sitter.

The Ascent

CROSSING THE THRESHOLD

Pause to reconnect with your intention. Why did you come here? What are you seeking? You are standing at a threshold, and once you step over, you can't turn back. Blow your prayer into your medicine or simply hold it in your hands for a minute. Let yourself settle, and when you are ready, welcome it into your body with an open heart.

SENSE PORTALS OPEN

Once the medicine begins to take effect, you may feel sleepy or relaxed, perhaps feeling an urge to stretch or yawn. The pupils of your eyes may dilate, mirroring your inner dilation. The apertures of your senses open as your perception of the outer world heightens; the strings of the guitar become sharper, the smell of burning cedar enters your cells, and the soft texture of your blanket is the coziest thing you've ever felt. Light seems brighter as your interior channels open wider, allowing more energy to flow through them.

You might feel like you're rising or sinking through atmospheric layers. Gravity shifts as you sense yourself hovering above the ground, humming, steam building as your rocket ship heads toward the sky. Alternatively, it can feel as though you are settling deeply into the earth below. You can feel a rush of emotions or begin to cry; some people call this phase "entering the rapids."

Whatever medicine you've taken is being absorbed into your bloodstream; spinning molecules are entering locks like keys, and biochemical reactions are beginning. Life force, prana, chi, or bioelectricity—whatever you call it—you'll notice that suddenly there is a lot more of it. You may feel tingly, effervescent, or anxious. Don't worry; it's just more energy entering your system.

Welcome the medicine into your body again and let yourself be like a river flowing into the ocean. Relax your muscles and mind, breathe into your belly, return to your intention, and trust the process. The elevation change is a phase, and you will soon find your cruising altitude.

WELCOMING DISSOLUTION

The walls soften, the ceiling droops, the internal steering wheel melts in your hands; physical reality loses its tone. Your familiar boundaries between self and world may become blurry, or you may lose touch with your sense of self altogether. You might feel like your center of gravity has moved to nowhere, or everywhere. Your mind can feel fluid and increasingly porous, with thoughts becoming glossy threads. Some people go straight to bliss. Others panic.

Think of the ego like scaffolding: a collection of habits, beliefs, and memories most people identify as their sense of self. With MDMA or low-dose ketamine you might perceive where your scaffolding is weak or needs repair. With classic psychedelics your scaffolding can become increasingly translucent. It may or may not entirely disappear, but it almost always loses its familiar solidity. You sense more space as the permeability of self is revealed. You might feel like you're dying or have done something terribly wrong. It's natural to feel shaky as familiar points of reference fade away.

The instinctual response is to fight what's happening and cling to the familiar. However, another option is to surrender to the dissolution, letting yourself become fluid. If you're willing to go with the experience, it will be less of a struggle. If you are with a guide, you can ask for reassurance; they will be familiar with this and encourage you through it, knowing it will pass.

Allow it all to swirl and twirl. Let yourself stop making sense and expand into the vastness. You might find that even without your familiar anchor points, you still feel completely "here." Some awareness or presence remains. Let yourself find a full-bodied "ah" and open into the rich space around you, becoming an ingredient in the cosmic soup. Let the room be your womb and let your mind unwind.

MORE MEDICINE?

You might have the chance to take a booster (another dose of medicine) at some point—something you should discuss with your guide ahead of time. They might ask: "Do you want more?" This can be a confounding question. Ask yourself: Do I want to go deeper, or is this depth just right? If you're writhing and wishing you could move through a portal you are stuck in, it can be helpful to take a bit more. If you're at the edge of your comfort zone and feeling afraid, perhaps it's better not to. You can always ask for a few minutes to decide, and instead of trying to use logic, let the question swirl around until you get a felt response. Let your body decide.

Navigating the Depths

As the intensified energy coursing through your body gains momentum, it can encounter stagnant areas. Like a river rising, the rushing water can hit against logjams of emotional debris. You might exhale a deep-held sadness or a rising frustration. You may feel nauseated as painful memories or tensions rise to the surface. While there may be stressful contractions and intense moments, they will pass.

SHAKING IT OUT

Your toes curl, and your feet twitch. The next thing you know, your knees are trembling, and if you let yourself, your legs start to shake. Or you feel a shiver starting in your shoulders and might think you're cold. Usually it's not your temperature. If you let yourself go with it, your shivers can evolve into full-on quaking.

Let your body follow its innate intelligence and unwind. By the time we're adults, many of us have been conditioned to contain our natural expression, so this can be surprising. But sometimes our bodies just need to shake. You might be shaking something out from long ago.

Let your body convulse like a gazelle that has escaped a lion. Quiver, tremble, vibrate from your head to your toes. Shake it out from the depths of your cells, your bones, your muscle fibers. Let yourself make sounds as needed. Don't hold it in. It wants to come out, and all you have to do is allow it. As much as you can, let go of concerns about how others might judge your expression. Guides and experienced sitters are used to this and expect it.

RELAXING WITH FEAR

Your animal body may react to the enormity of what you're experiencing, triggering memories of being out of control. You might feel things you prefer not to feel, like an involuntary clenching from your core, prickly, constricted, and shivering. Your heart rate may increase as blood pounds through your veins. You might feel like you're falling, that nothing is real, or fear that you'll be stuck in this state forever. Your fear might project onto the people around you, making them seem threatening or sinister.

If fear arises, ask yourself: Am I physically safe right now? It can be tempting to blame fear on the substance or the environment, or to judge the experience as bad. But even if you don't like what's happening, if you are indeed physically safe, see if you can refrain from seeking a cause. Relax with it as a pure experience and stay curious.

If things feel too intense, breathe deeply and rhythmically into your lower belly. If you're in an environment where it's appropriate, you can shout, roar, or even scream. Try pushing into the ground below you, or lying on your belly instead of your back. Most animals don't lie on their backs unless they're feeling playful and safe. Invoke any protective people, animals, or forces with whom you have a relationship. Imagine them and call on them.

If you're with a guide and have agreed to physical touch, reach out your hand or say, "I'm struggling," or simply, "Help!" Sometimes just asking shifts the energy. If you're alone, try rubbing your hands together, massaging your feet, or caressing your arms and face.

If fear persists, remind yourself: This is temporary. Don't mistake a portal for a destination. You are on a journey. Keep going.

PURIFICATION

As energy intensifies, tension or debris that has settled in the depths of your tissues often works its way toward the surface. It can feel like a toxic wave that makes you want to vomit, but it can also come out as sweat, tears, yelling, or even poop. You might feel dizzy or disgusted by a sticky heaviness.

Psychedelic medicines catalyze detoxification of the body, mind, and emotions. Obsessive thoughts, shame and bitterness, the mean things you tell yourself, and the memories that still sting can feel as though they are being drawn to the surface. Are these things actually coming out, or are you releasing the energy that's been bound up by them inside? Either way, let it out.

Allow yourself to purge in whatever way is needed. Get to the bathroom or, if you can, outside onto the earth. You can also purify by sitting up and breathing deeply, feeling your cells nourished by fresh oxygen. After any purge, cleanse yourself with cold water, a smudge of herbal smoke, or a refreshing spritz of rose or rosemary. Or step outside for some fresh air. Remember that some traditions refer to this as "getting well." It may feel awful in the moment, but your body is releasing what's been weighing it down.

EMOTIONAL STORMS

Emotions are wild and free; they don't want to be contained. Sometimes long-repressed emotional energy emerges like a beast that needs to howl. Anger can simmer or rush in like a firestorm. It needs to be released in its raw form, roaring or hissing. If you're in a setting where you can make noise, be as loud as you need for as long as you need.

At some point, you may feel caught in a loop of critical thoughts or painful feelings, like you're grinding gears or being ground through them. When your thoughts and emotions are amplified, you can feel like you're in a bottomless well. Like being caught in a rip current, fighting will exhaust you. If you can, zoom out and connect with the spaciousness in the room. You could try feeling both the intensity and the passing nature of it—an advanced practice.

Ask yourself: What am I being asked to feel right now? Is there any way I could open more to this wave? A few big belly breaths can help, as can asking for encouragement from your guide. If you can unleash your anger and get beneath it, you may discover sorrow or grief. Let yourself feel it and weep. If you catch a wave of joy or laughter, ride it as long as you can. Laughter is a locksmith, able to open stuck energy and unblock stagnation.

THE INFINITE VOID

You may find yourself somewhere new and unfamiliar, unsure which direction to follow. You might feel hollow, crushed, or completely cut off from sensation. It can seem like your momentum, your life force, has dissolved into smoke. You might arrive at a barren expanse that gives you nothing and makes no sense. You can scream into the infinite darkness, and there's no echo, no response.

This emptiness can feel terribly lonely and frightening, triggering an urge to escape or change it. You might be reliving memories from gestation, birth, or early experiences of being left alone in an incubator or crib. Many experienced psychedelic explorers and researchers believe such memories can reemerge in high-dose sessions, and the conversation is showing up in research settings.[1]

If an early memory is surfacing, it often needs to be fully experienced. Try changing your position: Uncross your limbs, lie on your belly, sit upright, or make subtle movements. Breathe deeply into your entire chest and expand in all directions.

Ask for strength from any wisdom beings, friends, or teachers you trust. Sometimes imagining their faces or saying their names brings support. If you have a guide, ask for help. Changing the atmosphere can help you move through a difficult passage. Opening a window or stepping outside with support can shift things.

Sometimes you try everything and nothing changes. The energy needed to move through this state may still be building, so try relaxing into the darkness. It's not about pushing: Sometimes the only way through is to experience the void fully. This phase may last longer than you want, but it will change, as all things do.

Revelations and Healing

RECEIVING VISIONS

Glowing neon ripples, shrouded figures, and rainbows weave into rivers of light, dripping into an endless abyss of darkness. Underwater reefs, pulsing mandalas, and enormous turquoise beings. Your childhood best friend, old lovers, unborn children, ancient grandmothers, and the cashier at your local grocery store, all morphing into one another in your mind's eye. Psychedelic visions can be sublime, horrific, or truly mind-boggling.

Although you may see the electric pink and green swirling fractals featured in movies, you might also see visions beyond your imagination. Sometimes you're catapulted back to childhood memories that were never fully integrated. You might see scenes of such beauty—an eagle taking flight, endless fields of wildflowers, rushing mountain streams—that they flood your heart with love. You might be immersed in disturbing visions—insects eating your decomposing body or beings watching you from the shadows. Or you may be shown shocking scenes of suffering—the devastation of war, senseless torture, or helpless beings crying for mercy.

When in realms of horror, a journey can feel overwhelming and prompt you to try to "change the channel." Pause and consider that you may be receiving this vision for a reason. Can you open yourself to the suffering or horror you're being shown and simply be with it? It's unlikely that anything you're seeing isn't happening somewhere on earth right now. This could be an invitation to connect with the broader human experience. You can ask: Why am I being shown this? What do I need to learn here? Let the vision unfold. Don't believe it or judge it. Just receive.

During his first ayahuasca journey, a friend began seeing horrific scenes of violence, ones he had not experienced himself. He allowed these to play out, though they were disturbing to witness. When they stopped, he felt an intense need to vomit and did. He later understood the vision was showing him how deeply societal violence had lodged into his body.

If what you're seeing feels beyond your capacity to endure, you can try to shift the vision. You can say, "Please, show me something else." Try returning to a prayer, mantra, or your intention. Ask for support if you have a guide.

REALIZATIONS

Insights fly like bolts of lightning, piercing veils of confusion and showing you the truth—or so it seems. There can be great pleasure in a deluge of understanding, in seeing how things are connected, or in realizing what you need to do. You might nod with each revelation, clapping at each new epiphany. How could you have missed this before? Your insights can seem so obvious in their moment of illumination, like a direct transmission.

Previously unconnected parts of your brain may be talking to one another for the first time. Maybe you suddenly realize you need to leave your job, have a tough conversation with an estranged cousin, or go on a pilgrimage to Japan.

Rather than proclaim victory, go farther. Ask: Show me what's below this. Keep peeling away the layers and see where the question takes you. Let new information come in; if it's meant to stay with you, it will. If it passes through your mind like a breeze, let it. If you have a guide, you can share your insights to be written down and read back to you later. If you're solo, you can record yourself and listen as part of your integration. Sometimes insights are unintelligible at first. You may understand them more clearly later.

Realizations may emerge that defy rationality yet feel more real than anything else. Remember: You're relating to your thoughts and emotions with unusual intensity, which doesn't necessarily make them more true. You don't have to do anything right now. Just let it all move through.

RECEIVING HEALING

During their journeys, many people experience direct healing—such as surgery or cellular reorganization—or receive guidance on what they need to do to heal. These experiences often transcend conventional scientific understanding.

I experienced this during a mushroom journey a year after completing chemotherapy when my risk for cancer recurrence was high. I brought an intention of asking to see if there was anything more I could do to stay cancer-free. During my journey, I felt my consciousness sink deep into my body. It was as though I had become tiny, looking at my body from the inside, examining my tissues and cells up close. Then two contrasting visions appeared: In one, I saw myself confused, tuned into another person's needs while neglecting my own, doing things I didn't want to do. I saw how this interaction permeated my mind and body with a dense fog, my cells becoming mushy. In the second vision, I was communicating clearly, saying no, and maintaining a clear boundary with the other person. The air brightened, and I saw my cells close up, a radiant vitality glowing around each one as they worked in harmony. "Cancer cells lack clear boundaries," the mushrooms explained. "Clarify the boundaries with people in your life and model it for your cells." While cancer is far more complex than relationship patterns alone, the guidance made sense and gave me something concrete to work with.

The Mystical Dimension

You may perceive the interconnectedness of all life. You might see how tree roots intertwine with networks of mycelia and remember that you are spinning on a sphere of water and rock, encircling a burning star, on a spiral dance through infinite space.

You might see how light refracts into the glowing matrix that manifests physical reality. The cosmos is dark and infinite but also brims with a radiance that can crack your heart wide open. You might hear the songs of your ancestors, celestial choirs, or a symphony of the stars. There can be a sense of divine rapture or ecstatic union as you encounter blazing winged angels who surround you with tenderness. You may find yourself surrounded by glowing star beings who anoint you as a galactic citizen or benevolent multiarmed deities who gather you into their embrace.

Many people come to psychedelic journeys seeking these exalted experiences. Yet there's a wide range of what could be considered mystical. Some are subtle and can affect you in mysterious ways. Experiencing communion with the nonhuman world—a fox, a hawk, an oak tree, or even your neighbor's cat—can connect you to the larger web of life.

In the face of magnificent beauty, it's possible to feel a wave of warmth and compassion. This compassion can melt every rigid knot in your mind, reminding you that ultimately, everything is all right. Overcome with devotion, you may feel the urge to fall on your knees in prayer or proclaim the exquisite grace of what you've been shown.

Being in such a state can be a gift; let the web of life envelop you. If you hear ethereal sounds—high-pitched bells or crystal flutes, for example—enjoy the music. It may be the playlist, but it might not be. Sometimes heaven sings to you.

If you experience cosmic love or splendor, the only thing to do is enjoy it. No need to grasp at rainbows; just let them bend into the far beyond. Immerse yourself in the majesty of these mystical dimensions, and let it seep deep into your bones so you can feel it vibrating within for days or weeks to come. The healing lies in allowing this ineffable beauty to permeate every level of your being.

PRIMAL AND SENSUAL ENERGY

You may feel a warmth pulsing through your body, like smoldering coals catching a flame. You might find your interest in the music increasing, feeling its rhythm in your hips, growing blissful or euphoric, your body wanting to move like a snake. You might feel an impulse to touch your skin, relishing its warmth and aliveness.

Revitalization of your pelvic area is common in psychedelic states. Sensual energy has been repressed for so long in so many cultures that when an opening appears and permission is present, it seizes the opportunity to liberate itself. While you might feel a charge building in specific parts of your body, this energy belongs to your entire body. This is primal energy reawakening, and labeling it solely as "sexual" minimizes its importance. Many traditions see the body as a bridge between heaven and earth, full of intelligent circuitry. You want to connect with all of your energy, sexual included. Feel the pleasure of this flowing magnetic force rushing through you. This awakening is healthy; primal energy may be the essence of health itself.

If the sensations are overwhelming, focus on your lower belly and breathe deeply. Many traditions consider the lower belly to be the location of your internal "storage battery" and the best place to draw in and contain energy. This primal awakening can be vulnerable and deserves protection. If a guide is present, their job is to make sure you can enjoy your own energy without involving themselves or making it relational or sexual.

The Return and Completion

THE CALL TO RETURN

Eventually, the moment will come when it's time to return to ordinary reality as your rocket ship descends to earth. This moment might appear as a rumbling in your stomach, a curiosity to sit up and look around, or a familiar question: What time is it? This question often signals that the scaffolding of your sense of self is reconstituting.

At this point, your body has metabolized most of the medicine, and you're returning to normal consciousness. Gently work your way out like a butterfly pushing out from the chrysalis. Transition slowly. There's no rush. Stay quiet and internally focused for as long as you need. You might not be ready to interact with anyone. Let the light in slowly, and allow your eyes to adjust. Everything you look at may appear beautifully saturated. Ideally, you're somewhere you can remain until all of you—your body, heart, and mind—are complete, since your return may not align with the clock.

RECONNECTING WITH OTHERS

You may feel the urge to connect with others, wanting to hold someone's hand or get a hug. This is a precious time to have gentle contact with whoever is present. It can be one of the most potent moments in your journey. You have the opportunity to reenter the world intentionally. Many of us missed out on a slow, warm welcome: Days in an incubator or overwhelmed parents may have made for a stressful introduction to life. This moment of emergence at the end of a journey can feel like rebirth, healing painful memories. The eyes of another gazing at you lovingly with full presence and encouragement as they welcome you back—this is healing balm for the human soul.

NOURISHMENT AND CELEBRATION

Your stomach may be growling, especially if you fasted before your journey. It's time to nourish and hydrate: Enjoy crackers, avocado, yogurt, nuts, fruit, tea, and electrolytes, or whatever you prefer. It's good to eat something salty and something sweet if you can. The first meal after a journey is incomparable. Enjoy the sensual pleasure of your taste buds, more awake than ever.

You have arrived at the time for toasting: Congratulations! If you feel a sense of accomplishment, luxuriate in it. You may feel ready to talk and connect, or you may prefer to stay quiet, completely still, right where you are. Stay where you are as long as necessary, provided you have food, water, and warmth. Only change locations when you're ready. Do whatever feels best. Sometimes your body is exhausted, but your mind isn't ready to return. Eat a nourishing meal, give yourself a night's sleep, and let everything unfold. If you find yourself in a tough spot, it's still good to rest. Sometimes the journey completes itself overnight.

CLOSING THE CIRCLE

If you called in any protectors, thank them and release them now. Close any portals you opened and formally complete the journey by blowing out a candle or saying a closing prayer.

Consider making a wish that anything beneficial from your experience ripples out to others in your life, or to all beings everywhere, multiplying the blessings you've received.

Though the formal ceremony is complete, this may be just the beginning. Relaxation, soulful gratitude, and unexpected revelations can continue to unfold for days or even years to come.

CHAPTER 9

Integration in Your Hands

You've emerged from your journey, and now you stand at a crossroads: You can turn right, to your familiar life with everything exactly where you left it. Or you can turn left, pausing to stay with the subtle sparks still pulsing through you, and sift through the glowing embers of your recent experience.

It's easy to compress back into the familiar version of yourself you know so well, but hold on! Allowing yourself to gently transition back to the normal pace of life is an act of self-kindness. Return at your own pace, not at a pace dictated by others. After all, you made a serious effort to travel into unfamiliar terrain and receive what it had to offer—why not linger with the experience, honoring your efforts and the medicine's gifts for as long as possible?

The flood of memories, unexpected insights, and sometimes startling visions that appear during a journey can exceed what you can process in real time, disrupting your usual sense-making and temporarily disorienting you. A psychedelic journey can take you to places so unfamiliar that it's like returning from the far side of the moon. You deserve to be welcomed back from this faraway land and listened to as you share everything you saw and everyone you met. Psychedelic integration is an act of inclusion, a way to bring relevant insights and lessons into your daily life.

Timing Matters: The Magic of Neuroplasticity

Through my own experience and years of helping others, I have seen the momentum of ingrained habits and the pull of familiar ways. Old patterns can return quickly. Realizations that were as clear as day during a journey can fade like a dream as daily life resumes. If you seek to heal or make substantial changes in your life, active participation and ongoing support will be required to sustain them.

Take advantage of the critical period, which lasts two days to four weeks, depending on which medicine you took. If your journey's intention was to explore habits or patterns causing pain in your life—such as chronic people-pleasing, unrelenting self-criticism, or excessive alcohol use—you might find some immediate relief afterward. You can thank your neuroplasticity and the shake-up that psychedelics give your brain for that. Unfortunately, the underlying causes of painful habits and behaviors usually don't completely resolve on their own. They require your attention.

A Brief History of Integration

In many spiritual traditions around the world, after an intense experience, a journeyer would typically visit an elder who would receive them, make sure they had fully "returned," and then help them shake off any debris. The elder might invite them into deeper reflection: What was learned, healed, or released? Sitting together, the elder would help them weave the threads of their experience back into their daily life.

Early psychedelic researchers and therapists in the United States saw the need for this aftercare support, realizing that lasting benefits didn't come from the session alone. Journeyers needed support to reflect on and work through their experiences. When psychedelic research resumed in the early 2000s, the Multidisciplinary Association for Psychedelic Studies, Johns Hopkins, the

Heffter Research Institute, and the Beckley Foundation all included preparation and integration sessions alongside the dosing session in their clinical trials.[1] The field had learned decades earlier that aftercare support is vital to lasting change.

Today, integration is understood to be a fundamental part of how psychedelic-assisted therapies heal. Guides who offer journey support almost always require one to three sessions, as do licensed facilitators working at healing centers in Colorado and Oregon.

Approaches to Integration

Some people criticize the practice of formal integration, pointing out that traditional communities rarely meet for scheduled integration sessions after group ceremonies. That may be true, but in traditional communities, daily life itself is integration, through regular conversations, meals, and shared child-rearing. Scheduled meetings aren't needed.

However, many people in the industrialized world don't live in tight-knit communities. In the isolation of a society centered around nuclear families, intentional integration meetings become useful. Next, I explore several ways to approach integration.

COMMUNITY SHARING CIRCLES

Group ceremonies often conclude with a sharing circle, during which each person is given a few minutes to share their experience. Sometimes solo or group artwork accompanies the verbal sharing. This is an excellent way to be listened to and mirrored by others while also hearing the struggles and victories of your fellow participants. Deeper bonding may arise from uncanny connections between people's experiences. One person's insight or challenge can resonate unexpectedly for someone else in the circle.

After a guided psilocybin ceremony in Oregon, one participant described a long conversation with his deceased younger brother, whom he was finally able to forgive for years of addiction and an early death. He realized his brother's actions were an attempt to self-medicate suffering he could never understand. The woman on his right broke into sobs. She had grappled all night with her relationship to her living sister, who was addicted to opiates. They were rarely in contact. She had been feeling angry, abandoned, and shut out for years. Hearing her fellow participant's story shifted something inside her. Maybe there was room for both her hurt and compassion for her sister. Moments like these show the power of shared witnessing.

The main limitation, however, is that everyone is spent. After a late night, an hour or so of sharing is about all people have in them. Participants don't receive individual attention, though many group facilitators offer an additional online integration meeting a week later. If that's not provided, consider self-organizing to meet as a group a few times.

While community sharing circles provide immediate support and deepening connection, you may want or need individualized attention to integrate your experience more thoroughly.

GUIDED INTEGRATION SESSIONS

If you have an individual journey with a guide, you will hopefully have one to three follow-up integration sessions scheduled. The more, the better. If you're returning from a solo journey or ceremony and want personalized support, you need to schedule these yourself. Aim to meet two or three times spread out over a few weeks.

The focus of these sessions should be on the content of your journey. When you meet, you can read your notes, share what came up—anger, grief, insights, visions, or memories—and ask for support with any changes you want to make. They can also help you reality-check any impulses that come up. Do you really want to leave your husband, move to Alaska, invest your savings in cryptocurrency, or start a church? Think of your journey like a dream: worth exploring, but not always meant to be taken literally.

If you have an ongoing psychotherapist or coach who is familiar with psychedelics and non-ordinary states of consciousness, they can be excellent support. Two to three sessions devoted to unpacking your journey are usually enough. The benefit of working with your regular therapist is that you can reflect on your journey throughout your work together and circle back for months to come.

You can also seek out a psychedelic integration specialist, sometimes called an integration coach or guide. They will likely include one or more techniques in their approach, such as somatic experiencing (SE), expressive arts, internal family systems (IFS), Jungian or depth work, or eye movement desensitization and reprocessing (EMDR). Whatever their approach, find someone comfortable with the nonlinear language of the deep psyche, which often expresses itself through feeling states and abstract images. The ideal qualities of an integration guide include good listening, creativity, and the capacity to wonder with you. They should ask what you saw, felt, and heard while treating your revelations with sincerity.

While your guide might feel protective or have strong opinions about what you should do, be careful that they don't overinterpret your experience or push an agenda. The point is for you to come to your own understanding, not adopt someone else's.

Beyond meetings with your guide, therapist, or ceremony group, you can tend to your integration on your own. Set aside time each morning to journal, share reflections with trusted friends or family, or look for a local or online integration circle.

Even if you receive a crystal-clear vision showing you how to approach something in your life, it will be up to you to take action. The support you need the day after a journey is often different from what you need two weeks later. The following timeline gives you a path to follow.

The Three Phases of Integration

LANDING AND REFLECTION: IMMEDIATE INTEGRATION

The first phase begins the morning after your experience and lasts up to three days.

The Day After

The day after your journey is best spent doing nothing. If that's a challenge, aim for half a day. Take it easy and recover in a relaxing and spacious environment. You may feel very spacey and "not all there" for a few days. This is normal and nothing to be alarmed by. It's best not to drive or operate machinery until you feel totally landed back in your body. Be gentle with yourself as you slowly return. Lie in a hammock, gaze at the sky, watch the waves, walk in a park, listen to the birds, or sit on the couch with a cup of tea. Take a hot bath or a sauna. Listen to gentle music and stretch. Skip the news and social media, and avoid staring at screens. Your brain is freshly neuroplastic, and your perception is still wide open. Stay as unplugged as you can.

Give yourself permission not to answer the phone or respond to texts and emails. Remember: You don't owe anyone a report of your experience. Resist the urge to jump into analysis, and instead stay curious and receptive as you absorb on deeper levels. Your journey will continue to land in you.

Grounding and Recovering

Focus on taking care of your body:

- Rest well.
- Drink plenty of fluids and electrolytes.
- Eat easy-to-digest nutrient-dense food; protein and root vegetables are best.
- Connect with friends and loved ones.
- Walk, hike, or move gently.
- Practice yoga, tai chi, or stretching.
- Get your bare feet on the earth or into the garden.
- Swim, bathe, or shower.

During this time, check in with yourself frequently. How do you feel in your body? What's your emotional state? Are you eating and sleeping well? If you're struggling to return to a balanced state, consider seeing an acupuncturist, bodyworker, or massage therapist you know and trust. Give yourself permission to do whatever you need to feel grounded: Eat macaroni and cheese, read a book, or watch a comedy.

While most people feel emotionally open or tender after a journey, some experiences require immediate professional attention. Seek professional psychiatric support if you experience manic or psychotic behavior, ongoing agitation or restlessness, rapid speech, suicidal or violent thoughts, or intense emotions that don't subside within three days.

Let It Steep

In our social media–saturated world, the impulse to share everything immediately is strong. It's as if nothing is meaningful without external validation and existence has become contingent on visibility. You may want to exclaim to the world, "Mushrooms helped me stop smoking," or "LSD showed me that love is the only true force in the universe." But immediate sharing can give something away before it's fully absorbed. Healing and revelation are worth celebrating, but keep them private for a while. Let your realizations steep and infuse you with their power. Listening to music from your journey can help the steeping process.

Begin to Reflect

Sometimes meaning-making can take you away from the potency of what is cooking inside, so wait until you feel ready. Sit down with your pen and journal, and record as much as possible while it's fresh. You may doubt your capacity to recall everything, but as soon as you put pen to paper, the words often pour out. Rather than typing on a device, try writing your reflections by hand. This allows for a clearer flow from mind to page.

Beware of the tendency to judge with questions like: Was it good? Did it work? Do I want to do this again? Instead, think of your writing as a fresh transmission from the other side. Let your words be poetic or abstract if that feels authentic, or write out your experience scene by scene, like the script of a play. Don't worry about remembering things sequentially. Just let loose and write. If you find yourself staring at a blank page, here are a few prompts:

- What did you see, hear, or feel?
- Were there any recurring images, symbols, or beings?
- What happened?
- And then what happened?
- Were there any challenging parts? What were they?
- What surprised you?
- What parts were most meaningful?
- Did you receive any insight or guidance?
- Is there anything you are left wondering about?

If journaling isn't your thing, drawing, dancing, or making a collage can work just as well. Get some pastels or markers and draw out everything you saw and felt. A mandala is a beautiful way to draw out what's inside: Take a large piece of paper, draw a circle on it, then start filling it in intuitively, and see what emerges. If you're a musician, let sound come through. There might be a song right now waiting to be sung.

Stay Human

An increasing number of people are using ChatGPT and other AI tools to analyze their psychedelic journey notes. You may receive an intellectually coherent analysis this way, but you'll miss the deeper integration that comes from wrestling with the mystery of it yourself. The work of sitting with the raw content of your journey is alchemical, inviting you to forge a relationship with what emerged. You don't want to miss this by outsourcing it. If you must use AI tools, give yourself at least a week to write, draw, and reflect independently before seeking external analysis. Steeping in your own messy unfolding is where the deeper integration happens.

CONTEMPLATION AND ACTION

The second phase of integration takes place over the three to fourteen days following your journey. For most medicines this is the heart of the neuroplastic window. Use this time to contemplate deeper meanings. From there, think through any actions you want to take and how to find the support you need.

Don't rush or let others rush you to interpret your experience before you're ready. If someone pushes you to describe what happened, you might feel blank, confused, or emotionally overwhelmed. This means you aren't ready to translate what you went through into words yet, and that's okay. Your nervous system needs more time to settle. If they don't notice your need to slow down, you can pause them and let them know.

Sharing and Meaning-Making

A good first step is sharing your journey notes or drawings with your guide or a friend, along with any meanings beginning to surface. Read your story out loud, slowly and lovingly, or share any art you've created. If your facilitator took notes, listen as they read them back to you. If you want to share something with a friend or family member who is skeptical about psychedelics, you can simply say, "I had a dream. . . ."

Images, sensations, memories—your experience may seem like a tangle of colored yarn. Follow the threads that call to you, pulling each strand apart to see its length, color, and texture. Your intention now serves as a key to decode your experience. How might the visions or messages you received be a response to it?

Questions for Contemplation

- Which images or symbols that you saw feel significant now?
- Are there any big emotions still present in your body? If so, what might they be telling you?
- Have any patterns in your life become clearer? What might you want to work on?

- What was the central message of your journey, and how might it be in response to your intention?
- Are there any realizations you'd like to translate into your daily life?
- Does any part of your experience feel incomplete? What might help it feel resolved?

Taking Action

Therese, a newly retired accountant, sought out a guided mushroom journey, hoping for a vision for the next stage of her life. At the peak of her journey, she felt herself drawn up into the atmosphere and looking down at the earth. She saw vivid scenes of suffering—burning forests, polluted oceans, people pushed off their homelands. She wept for two days afterward, feeling powerless in the face of what she saw. At her first integration session, her guide asked if her visions could be a response to her intention. Therese realized she was being guided to get involved in her community, a place where she had the power to help. She began volunteering at a local nonprofit, delivering food to families in her town.

The following questions can help you move from understanding the themes of your experience to taking action:

- Is it time to bring more joy, color, play, or pleasure into your life? How could you do this?
- Is there a spiritual practice, therapy, exercise routine, new path of study, or pilgrimage you want to pursue?
- Is there any activism or community service you'd like to get involved in?
- Is there an apology, confession, or request you need to make? A letter to write? A ritual to perform?
- Is there someone you need to say goodbye to? If they are no longer living, consider writing them a letter and reading it to someone else, then burying or burning it.
- Is it time to look for a new job or end a relationship?
- Is it time to seek support for an addiction that's causing you or others pain?

Now contemplate what the first small steps might be. Trust the natural impulses that arise from within, but if you're considering a significant life change, such as quitting your job or getting married or divorced, let it simmer for two weeks and discuss it with a trusted guide, therapist, or mentor.

Grace, a first-generation American, worked eighty-hour workweeks at a tech startup and struggled with regular migraines and digestive problems. She came to me for integration support six months after an MDMA journey with friends. She had realized something crucial that she couldn't shake: Her hard-working immigrant parents had given her the best education they could, yet their constant pressure on her to make more money and start a family was making her sick. Once she saw how her symptoms were connected to the stress of trying to meet their expectations, Grace knew she needed to say something. It took a few more months for her to feel ready, but finally, she spoke with them. Though the conversation was hard, Grace was able to set a boundary. Their relationship was strained temporarily, but her physical symptoms slowly improved. She was learning to prioritize her well-being over her parents' approval.

Sometimes what you're being asked to do is surprisingly simple. One client's journey intention was to step into greater service in the world. She had anticipated a vision telling her to move across the globe and join a humanitarian cause. In the end, the homework she got was to exercise more and to start calling her mom back. She decided to start there.

RETROSPECTION AND NOURISHMENT: ONGOING INTEGRATION

This third phase begins about two weeks after your journey and can extend for years.

Tending the Revelations

Continue writing about your experience and nurture any artistic expression that emerges. Keep learning about the symbols or images you saw. If an animal appeared to you, look for photos, documentaries, or books about that creature. Do the same if you had a vision of a historical person or place. Trust that the vision is speaking to something deep inside you and that it's worth following the thread. Sometimes a particular song from your journey can become an inner anthem.

Layers Reveal Over Time

When you receive instruction from a wisdom teacher—whether in human, plant, mushroom, or chemical form—you can only take in so much at a time. Months or even years later, reading your journey notes, looking at drawings, or revisiting a playlist can bring you right back to the experience. You might discover a new layer to process. Often, it's only in retrospect that we understand the deeper aspects of what we were shown.

Raymond, whom I worked with for a few months after an ayahuasca ceremony, told me he had walked out on the deck during the evening and stared into a grove of redwood trees. After a few minutes, he turned and asked one of the assistants, "Have the trees always been dancing?" Though his ceremony revealed many things, it was the dancing trees that stayed with him. He began taking long walks every Sunday at a local reservoir, finding a spot to sit among the trees. Every other time we would meet, he'd return to this simple discovery, smiling with wonder: "I've been on earth for six decades, and I never knew the trees were dancing."

Periodically it can be helpful to reflect on your life. Has anything shifted? Have your relationships transformed? Can you track any of it back to your journey and your intention?

Not Everything Requires Integration

Despite my enthusiasm, I want to acknowledge that not every experience requires active follow-up work. Sometimes a single moment during a journey can land so completely that no further processing is needed.

Jacob, an older friend with decades of psychedelic experience, recounted a vision that changed him. At the time, he was a stressed father of two young children and often yelled at his kids in moments of exasperation. During a high-dose LSD session, he suddenly found himself looking up through the eyes of a small child as an enormous, angry man towered over him, yelling. He curled up and trembled, terrified.

Jacob emphasized this was not a personal memory; his own father had been gentle and patient. He viscerally understood how damaging his outbursts were and rarely raised his voice at his children again. No follow-up was needed.

Sometimes the medicine does the teaching or the healing, and nothing needs to be done afterward. The key is learning to distinguish between experiences that need only to be received and those that are asking for your time and dedication to be embodied.

When You Need Extra Care

LIFE-CHANGING VISIONS

I met with a client who came for support after a group mushroom ceremony. At our first meeting, he told me he had a vision of moving his family to Portugal. He was fed up with the United States, and this was the clarity he'd been waiting for. He was planning to give two weeks' notice at his job within a few days. I asked if he knew anyone in Portugal. "No." Did he have a job that could transfer? "Not sure." Had they looked into visa requirements? "No, not yet." It was clear he had more research to do, so I encouraged him to keep his job and take another two weeks to consider the move before making any drastic changes. He nodded. "Fine. That's what my wife told me too."

Psychedelic journeys can reveal areas of your life that are stagnant or overripe. You might finally see that your struggling marriage has no future or that your job is making you sick. Or, after years of dreaming about moving to a monastery, you suddenly feel ready. A repressed part wakes up and is hell-bent on shaking things up—now! You emerge with the energy and ambition to take the leap you've been waiting for.

If the change doesn't affect anyone else and gives you more health or freedom, go for it. Declutter your closets. Delete social media. Go vegetarian. Pour out the vodka or throw out the cigarettes. Cancel the third date if you know it's going nowhere. However, for bigger decisions, especially those that impact others, give yourself time to let the impulse settle. Talk your ideas through with a few friends, your guide, or an integration coach.

MEMORIES OF ABUSE

Psychedelics can bring you into experiences beyond your direct life history, like visiting other places and times or seeing images while feeling their impact viscerally in your body. Sometimes, visions of emotional, physical, or sexual abuse can emerge unexpectedly. Are these literal memories or symbolic visions?

It's worth knowing that visions can sometimes draw from the collective unconscious, ancestral trauma, or symbolic representations of emotional pain rather than literal events from your life. Some practitioners believe we can access our ancestors' memories, passed down through generations. This doesn't make a vision less real or important—it still needs attending to—but understanding that it might not be from your personal history can provide relief if the images don't match anything you or your family members remember.

Either way, you should not be alone with this question. Whether literal or symbolic, these visions are asking for your attention. Find someone experienced with childhood trauma to help you work through what you saw and felt. If your guide is not a specialist in this area, they should help you find a therapist trained to work with sexual abuse.

If they are true memories, the healing may begin with righteous anger and disgust. With proper support, the rage often moves toward grief and sorrow. Let these feelings emerge organically as you move through them at your own pace.

You may want to confront the perpetrator if you believe the memories are accurate, but move slowly. At times, confrontation is the right thing to do—both to prevent additional abuse and because confronting the abuser may be part of your healing. However, confrontation can also bring new pain, such as family members who don't believe you or an abuser who denies the allegations. This doesn't mean you shouldn't confront someone. It means you should seek a skilled trauma therapist to help you decide the best path forward and stay by your side through whatever unfolds.

FEELING INCOMPLETE OR HAVING "NO EXPERIENCE"

If you feel like you came out of your journey lacking resolution, the work might not be complete. You may feel anxious, depressed, or physically sick. You may also feel stuck or "out of it." You might need help from an experienced guide or integration coach to work through where you're stuck. Some people find that gentle guided breathwork can help move you through a phase like this.

Another challenging experience is making sense of having had no experience at all. Sometimes you prepare thoroughly, take the medicine at the right dose, and open yourself to the experience—and nothing happens. This can be maddening. Is it biochemical? Psychological? Nobody knows why, but it happens. Ask yourself: Could this be showing me something about my relationship with expectations and disappointment? If you weren't on medications or supplements that could have interfered with the medicine, it's possible that your lackluster response was a one-time event, and it's worth giving it another shot.

It's possible that in some mysterious way, your experience was what your psyche or soul needed that day. Pay attention to any subtle clues you may have picked up: the sensations in your body, the emotions you felt, the thoughts in your head. These can act as a vivid mirror even when there are no fireworks.

THE DIFFICULT JOURNEY

As discussed in chapter 2, the infamous "bad trip" encompasses a range of experiences: fear, panic, disorientation, rage, or overwhelm. It can include frightening visions, traumatic memories, looping thought patterns, believing that you're dying, or intense physical sensations like a racing heartbeat, headache, nausea, or vomiting.

Facilitators may respond more or less skillfully, but intense feelings are part of the package with non-ordinary states of consciousness. These same experiences can also happen during intensive meditation retreats, breathwork, and vision quests. Struggle doesn't equate to failure.

If you have an experience like this, seek support from a practitioner experienced in psychedelic integration. If you can't find someone, look for local or online integration circles, where experienced journeyers may offer helpful insights. Most importantly, reach out to emotionally supportive people in your life.

What makes a trip "bad" isn't the difficulty itself; it's the feeling of not being held well by your community afterward. When we go through challenging experiences, we need to be surrounded by caring humans.

⌘ ⌘ ⌘

A psychedelic journey, as extraordinary as it can be, is limited in how much change it can create on its own. You have to meet it halfway. This requires your time and attention. It takes courage to embark on a journey into the unknown and to navigate the uncertainty of how new information might affect your life. And it takes ongoing determination and creativity to change routines and relationships—and to become who you came here to be.

Regardless of what type of journey you have—challenging, transformative, or somewhere in between—every experience deserves your attention and care over the days, weeks, and months afterward. This is your precious opportunity to honor what emerged and consciously choose how it shapes your life moving forward.

Whether you pursue integration within a community, with a guide, or on your own, and whether you follow my suggestions or do it entirely your own way, giving yourself this gift means intentionally coming into a more intimate relationship with yourself. This gift will serve you in ways that extend far beyond the journey. Be careful, though: Integration can be a gateway drug to a more awake and contemplative way of life.

CHAPTER 10

Navigating Power with a Psychedelic Guide

What good is consciousness without conscience?

Frank Herbert, author of the science fiction novel *Dune,* wrote, "Power attracts pathological personalities. It is not that power corrupts, but that it is magnetic to the corruptible."[1]

Like any formidable technology, psychedelic-assisted healing has its shadow side. The shadow refers to a collection of hidden, denied, or repressed impulses and characteristics that the conscious part of the psyche refuses to acknowledge. It contains everything we intentionally hide or unconsciously avoid. Ignoring the shadow gets you into trouble. In Carl Jung's words, "By not being aware of having a shadow, you declare a part of your personality to be nonexistent. . . . If you get rid of qualities you don't like by denying them, you become more and more unaware of what you are."[2]

When you add psychedelics to the mix, the denial of the shadow can become amplified and dangerous. As Stan Grof famously said, "LSD and other psychedelics function more or less as nonspecific catalysts and amplifiers of the psyche."[3] This amplification doesn't stop at your internal experience; it extends to your interactions with your guide. Every word uttered, every movement made, and every emotional shift can have a disproportionate impact.

Think of it as therapy on steroids. You don't even have to consume the substance to receive the amplification effect. When one person takes a psychedelic at a high enough dose, anyone sensitive in the room can feel expanded too, just from breathing the same air. This magnifies everything—the glowing, benevolent aspects of a person's character as well as their unconscious patterns. Understanding how amplification intensifies suggestibility and psychological projections will help you navigate potential tangles.

In this realm of healing, shadow aspects, especially those relating to the facilitator-client relationship, are under-discussed. Because this work largely operates in a legal gray area, some practitioners believe they can do whatever they please. Without agreed-upon standards or enforceable regulations, best practices are sometimes ignored. The more aware you are of the range of behavior you may encounter, from impeccable to sloppy to dangerously negligent, the better equipped you are to respond when something feels off.

The Asymmetry of Power

We all have areas where we naturally hold more authority and those where we defer to someone else. When we share power equally, as with a friend or colleague, our interactions can feel like a dance; sometimes we lead, and at other times, they do. These dynamics are always present, and it feels good when power is balanced and shared well.

Other times, power is inherently asymmetrical. When you go to a doctor, they decide whether to order the blood tests or scans needed for a correct diagnosis. If they try to save time or cut costs and don't order the proper tests, you could receive an incorrect diagnosis. Asymmetrical relationships exist when there is a considerable difference in education or expertise, age, economic power, racial privilege, or disability status—any aspect of identity that affects how we relate to others.

When the person with more power makes decisions with the vulnerable person's well-being in mind, they are likely to provide the best outcome. When they make decisions with their own interests in mind, damage can result.

Kylea Taylor, author of *The Ethics of Caring* and *Peer Consultation Groups and Ethical Awareness Tools for Psychedelic Practitioners*, uses the term "Responsible Party" to refer to "the person who is responsible for the care and protection of a person who is in an extra-ordinary state of consciousness; the caregiver who prioritizes the cared-for other person's best interests."[4] In psychedelic work, your guide is the Responsible Party.

WHO SEEKS POWER?

Psychedelics hold tremendous power. They attract people who want to help others; many guides working in this field are dedicated to the people they serve and value ethical integrity. However, psychedelic medicines and guide work also attract those seeking influence and those who crave admiration or even guru-like devotion. Providing potent substances that dramatically shift consciousness, rendering clients vulnerable—often with no one else in the room—gives someone an unparalleled position of authority.

People with narcissistic tendencies are often drawn to working as psychedelic guides. They may be charismatic, conduct breathtaking ceremonies, or be stellar musicians, often attracting admiration, even idolization. Yet these talents do not ensure they have the maturity and conscience required to work intimately with people's emotional worlds.

Some psychedelic guides think of themselves as spiritual teachers, empowered to challenge taboos, claiming it's necessary to help others push through "limiting beliefs." While expanded states can reveal our interconnectedness and show us transcendent dimensions of reality, guides who spend extensive time in non-ordinary states sometimes lose sight of the distinction between spiritual reality and everyday reality. This can lead to what's called "spiritual bypassing": a tendency to focus on transcendent oneness while dismissing earthly consequences, often showing up as sloppy behavior and a lack of empathy for human vulnerability.

Some guides operate in an "intuitive style," assuming their good intentions are enough to protect their clients from harm, without understanding the complexities of power dynamics or consent. While these guides may not be intentionally crossing boundaries, they may be unconsciously mishandling the vulnerability that psychedelic sessions create. Working with a distracted or neglectful guide is frustrating, but if you have a history of childhood neglect or abuse, experiencing neglect in a non-ordinary state can reactivate painful wounds. Similarly, a guide's limited relational skills—scattered attention, weak boundaries, poor communication—can create confusion even when there's no malicious intent.

A mature psychedelic facilitator with solid personal power doesn't need their clients' validation to feel secure. When guides are self-reflective and committed to healthy relationships, they're far more likely to use their position responsibly and handle challenges skillfully. They take feedback seriously and work to repair any ruptures that take place. They know that illuminating what lies in the shadow can humble us and inspire growth.

HOW POWER IMBALANCES SHOW UP

The same guide who helps you heal can also cause you harm. These aren't mutually exclusive. People want to think in binary terms: Someone is either good or bad, safe or dangerous. But a guide can offer you genuine healing in one moment and cross a boundary in the next. This complexity is one of the biggest obstacles to recognizing when something is off. If someone helped you break through a lifelong pattern, how can they also be the person who violated your trust? And yet both can be true.

When power dynamics are unhealthy, especially in inherently asymmetrical relationships, there can be a subtle feeling that you're supposed to act a certain way or that you shouldn't do something you want to do. You suddenly feel young, as though you're trying to please your guide and be the "good client." Alternatively, you may feel rebellious and determined to resist any guidance they offer. These feelings can be challenging to articulate as the dynamics that surround them often cause confusion.

Sometimes a guide's misuse of power is obvious. For example, right before taking the medicine, you decide you want a lower dose, but your guide insists on the higher dose. Fearing their disappointment, you comply, only to feel uneasy and nauseated for hours.

Misuse of power can also be more subtle and harder to notice. Your guide's need to be seen as wise or spiritually gifted can quietly shift the focus of your journey from your inner experience to their interpretation of it. Say you're weeping about your father's death toward the end of a journey. Your guide announces they sense your father's spirit in the room, asking you for forgiveness. You nod, grateful for their intuitive gift, while another part of you feels uncomfortable. You still have righteous anger to process and aren't ready for forgiveness. What seems good-hearted becomes more about your guide showcasing their abilities or imposing spiritual authority.

A boundary overstep like this can appear gentle and well-intentioned, and you might not recognize it until much later, if at all. This is particularly insidious when a guide genuinely believes they're helping. Their conviction that they're doing good can make their influence even more persuasive when you're in a suggestible state. There are no warning signs of malicious intent because there is no malicious intent. The guide is living in a reality where their behavior makes perfect sense, which makes it harder for you to trust your own discomfort.

SOCIOCULTURAL POWER DYNAMICS

These dynamics become more complex when we acknowledge the sociocultural forces that become amplified in psychedelic therapy. We live in cultures rife with hierarchies based on age, education, skin color, gender, economic status, and other arbitrary distinctions. If a guide fails to address these underlying dynamics explicitly, social hierarchies can seep into the healing space unconsciously.

Ema, a young Japanese American woman, came to me for integration support after a series of ketamine-assisted therapy sessions with an older, wealthy, white female guide. She described how, as the medicine took effect and her defenses softened, she'd become even more deferential than usual. Her cultural conditioning to respect her guide as a successful elder was intensified by the substance. Over the weeks, her guide became increasingly confident and directive during their integration sessions. Ema found herself going along with guidance that didn't feel right.

The medicine amplified preexisting power dynamics for both of them: Ema's cultural tendency to defer and her guide's unconscious assumption that Ema's politeness meant agreement. Without explicit discussion of these dynamics beforehand, the psychedelic space became a place where social hierarchies were magnified rather than examined.

WHAT YOU CAN DO ABOUT POWER DYNAMICS

It's not your job to educate your guide about racism, economic inequality, gender bias, or any other power differential affecting your therapeutic relationship. It's your guide's job, as the Responsible Party, to educate themselves.

But what if your guide is oblivious to the power differential showing up between you? Should you walk away? Not necessarily. If you feel a strong connection with them, ask for a conversation to talk through what happened. They might take full accountability and apologize. We all have blind spots, and we all make mistakes. Feel free to give feedback. A mature and humble practitioner will appreciate your feedback, listen closely, and be willing to learn something new to support you. If they're unwilling to meet you halfway, it's your prerogative to walk away and seek professional services elsewhere.

Anyone who calls themselves a healer should know how to have reparative conversations and be able to take accountability for their mistakes or missteps. They should also understand how systemic dynamics—racism, economic inequality, gender bias—perpetuate power imbalances and contribute to suffering.

Navigating Suggestibility

Can you remember something an adult told you when you were young that has stayed with you? At five, my mom told me, "No matter what anyone's circumstances are, they deserve to be treated well. Always share food when you can." Her words positively shaped my worldview. But what if the words you heard were hateful or full of fear? What is said to you while in a wide-open psychedelic state can shape your beliefs just as deeply.[5]

Suggestibility begins before you take the medicine. Everything in the room where you journey can influence your experience—from the elephant-headed god Ganesh to the whimsical mushroom poster and the Virgin Mother on the altar. If possible, visit your journey space beforehand. Do you want your guide to remove anything? Do you want to bring your own statue or art? If they don't oblige, decide what you can live with. It's your consciousness that will be wide open, not theirs.

Music is equally influential. A good guide will spend considerable time crafting a unique playlist for you, gathering songs and lyrics they anticipate will resonate with your inner state. However, if lyrics clash with your experience or are disturbing, they can leave you feeling disoriented or violated. If this concerns you, tell your guide what music you enjoy and specify any songs, genres, or artists you'd prefer not to hear. You can ask about bringing your own playlist, though many guides are hesitant about this. Your favorite songs might not work as you expect in an expanded state. The question of who controls the music touches on a deeper question: Do you feel safe enough to let go of control and trust your guide's expertise? If not, discuss this beforehand.

Your guide's comments and nonverbal communication can also influence your consciousness. Their influence might be obvious through the prayer they recite at the beginning of your journey or their repeated questions about the abuse you told them you "might" want to discuss. It can be less obvious through their raised eyebrows when you mention the stimulant addiction you have struggled with for years, or an offhand warning about malevolent aliens or dark entities you might encounter.

Suggestibility extends into your integration sessions as well. Does your guide direct meaning-making toward their preferred therapeutic outcomes, their spiritual cosmology, or their desire for referrals, even if they aren't fully aware of it? If your guide is opinionated and intent on expressing their views, they can have a marked impact on you. This is why you should ask them about their worldviews before working together. Suggested questions are included in appendix B, "Questions to Ask Before Choosing a Psychedelic Guide."

The question isn't whether a facilitator will influence your experience; they will. That's their job. The question is whether they influence your experience in a way that serves your intention. You're hiring this person to spend intimate time with your undefended psyche, so ensure you're with someone mindful of their words and actions. Choose someone who will center your intentions and welcome your unique interpretations, regardless of their personal beliefs.

A Hall of Mirrors: Navigating Projections

Until we unpack the past, the human mind acts like a projector, casting unresolved history onto the present. When something stirs a charged memory, we can find ourselves projecting our unmet needs, fears, or resentment onto the people around us. We can also project adoration, love, and yes, sexual attraction. The vulnerable, intimate nature of psychedelic healing work, combined with the long hours together, intensifies this process.

The phenomenon of projection is often at the root of complicated and damaging relationships with psychedelic facilitators. A basic understanding of how psychedelics amplify this phenomenon, known in the field of psychology as *transference,* can help you navigate tangles and avoid harm. Carl Jung described it this way:

> Unconscious contents are invariably projected first upon concrete persons and situations. Many projections can ultimately be integrated back into the individual once he has recognized their subjective origin; others resist integration, and although they may be detached from their original objects, they thereon transfer themselves to the doctor.[6]

In other words, we often project our unresolved feelings onto others. Some projections we can recognize and reclaim; others simply shift to whoever is closest, often the person trying to help us.

HOW PROJECTIONS SHOW UP

Sharing your innermost feelings, fears, and fantasies might lead you to develop a sense of gratitude toward your guide. As you appreciate their patience, you may grow to admire them. After receiving the attention you were starved for as a child, you might find yourself wanting to thank them profusely or embrace them.

Projections work both ways. Like therapists, guides can project unconscious feelings onto clients too, a phenomenon called *countertransference*. For example, if you view your guide as powerful and brilliant and regularly praise them, the flattery may meet their unconscious longing to be admired. They might begin to see you as the adoring student they've been waiting for and treat you with extra care. The relationship is no longer primarily about your healing; it now includes meeting their needs as well.

At other times, projection can come from the guide, such as when they play "the rescuer." A guide working with a young trauma survivor might feel protective parental impulses, acting beyond their agreement: offering extra sessions, sending job opportunities, or maintaining open text communication outside sessions. These good-natured gestures would be appropriate from a friend or family member, but that's not what the client hired them for. These gestures can slide into the realm of a "dual relationship," in which a client is expected to relate to their guide in multiple ways without clear boundaries. If you are invited to assist them in ceremony or babysit their children, does it mean you will get better care as a client, or worse? This complicates and reduces the potency of the healing contract.

PROJECTIONS CAN HELP US HEAL

Projections themselves do not pose a problem; in fact, they can be a valuable part of the healing process. When a skilled guide tracks them with objective curiosity and reflects them back to you, it can help increase self-awareness. At the very least, a guide's job is to be aware of this phenomenon and understand the hall of mirrors that projections create. They should try not to get caught up in it, but if they do, it's their job to realize it quickly, seek supervision, and stick to the professional agreement, even when dynamics become complicated. Listen to your gut and seek another perspective if you feel something is off.

Navigating Touch, Consent, and Boundaries

PHYSICAL TOUCH

In psychedelic healing, touch can be profoundly reassuring: a hand on your shoulder, a steady grip when you're shaking, a blanket placed over you. The body often needs contact to feel safe, and skilled guides know how to use touch as part of the healing.

But your body belongs to you, and the space around it belongs to you. If someone wants to touch you, they need to ask for your consent, ideally well before you've consumed mind-altering medicine. Consent practices are critical to maintaining a safe and empowering atmosphere, yet they're often left out of the conversation, perhaps because asking can feel awkward or break the flow of the moment. That's not a good enough reason. When it comes to healing work, asking permission is a professional obligation.

While many people feel neutral about touch, or think they do, others are highly sensitive to it because of their cultural background or past boundary violations, including sexual abuse. A guide should discuss beforehand the types of physical contact they might offer you during your journey. They should be well-versed in best practices regarding consent and able to discuss the benefits and risks of touch, providing you with all the information you need to decide what kind of support you want.

Healers in certain traditional cultures may use physical touch during ceremonies—applying oils, herbs, or smoke to remove harmful energies or strengthen your body—and may not ask your consent beforehand. If this concerns you, seek guides who center consent and actively prioritize your boundaries, or choose settings within a cultural context you're familiar with. Even in traditional cultures, contact should never be sensual or sexual in nature during a healing ceremony. That is a violation anywhere. I address sexual boundary violations directly in the next chapter.

THE ULYSSES CONTRACT: HONORING AGREEMENTS

During Ulysses's decade-long mythical voyage through the Mediterranean Sea, his ship neared an island inhabited by sirens: mesmerizing creatures whose songs promised to reveal all the secrets of the earth. However, the sirens' song was also known to enchant sailors, who would abandon their ships and die under the spell. Ulysses devised a plan to hear their song safely. He had his crew tie him tightly to the mast, instructing them to plug their own ears with wax. As soon as he heard the sirens' song, he begged his crew to untie him. Fortunately, his men stayed the course until they were beyond the island.

The Ulysses contract refers to a self-binding agreement made while you are in a clear state of mind for a future when you won't have the same capacity for wise decision-making.[7] In psychedelic facilitation, it can be used to steer a guide's actions regarding physical contact. If a client says during preparation that they do not want physical contact, the guide remains true to the original agreement. Even if the client changes their mind once they are altered, pleading with the guide to hold their hand, the original request stands. When this change of mind happens, it can be challenging, but this keeps everyone safe until the client returns to normal consciousness.

Not all psychedelic facilitators agree with the Ulysses contract. Some believe it can be harmful to deny a client touch when they ask for it, regardless of their state of mind. It's true that it can hurt to suddenly feel young and tender, wish for a hand to hold, and be told no. However, honoring the original agreement is the best practice here. Feelings of rejection can be worked through during an integration session, and agreements can be adjusted for future journeys.

And if you do give consent for physical contact before a journey, you can change your mind at any time. You can hold your guide's hand for five seconds and decide it's not what you want after all. No means no, whether you are sober or expanded. If there is any physical touch, it should always be for you, not to satisfy your guide's need to feel useful or meet their own desire for contact.

SURRENDER

"Surrender" is often touted as a goal in therapeutic psychedelic work. However, there is confusion about what surrender means. It does not mean complying with a guide's preferences or agenda. True surrender is about opening to the expanded state and allowing the medicine to work. If you're encountering resistance or trying to control your experience, there's likely a good reason. A skilled guide will help you explore your resistance rather than pressuring you to override it. They might ask: "What can I do to help you feel more comfortable right now?" rather than insisting you relax. Surrender isn't about giving up your agency. It's about opening to your experience on your terms, at your pace.

At some point you may want to intentionally work with your resistance, but this requires your consent and a conversation beforehand. I worked with an experienced client who asked me to play Guns N' Roses during his mushroom journey. He didn't like their music; in fact, he hated it. But they had been his mom's favorite band, the soundtrack of his painful childhood. He wanted to confront the revulsion the music brought up in him. When he first heard the music, he was tense. Then he began to cry. After two songs, I changed the music, but he told me to put it back. We listened to hard rock together for the next hour while he wept. He was surrendering, by choice, to something difficult—not to me. That's the distinction that matters.

In some traditional settings and ceremonies, the guide will follow a structure of songs, prayers, and other ritual elements that they aren't willing or able to change in response to your preferences or discomfort. There may be drums, rattles, or long intense songs. This isn't an agenda; it's a structured ceremony that proceeds according to tradition, whether or not you like it. As long as you are physically safe and your boundaries are not being violated, it's best to patiently endure the ceremony until it's complete, respecting the cultural context you are in.

Understanding power dynamics, projections, and consent is essential, but knowledge alone isn't enough. Ultimately you must take responsibility for your own discernment throughout the process.

Your Responsibility

It is your job to bring your best discernment to the process of choosing a guide and to stay aware of your own tendency to project perfection or dismiss concerning behaviors. Stay alert if any troubling signs start to emerge before a scheduled journey. Pause and ask questions at any time if something feels off.

It helps to stay respectfully businesslike when paying for a service. Are you receiving what you came for? If not, address it, and if it doesn't shape up, maybe it's time to walk away. It's good to check in with yourself frequently and take the pulse of any healing relationship. Are your comfort and trust growing? Are small shifts in the right direction beginning to appear?

If you're ever uncertain about a guide's behavior, seek the perspective of someone outside the relationship—a therapist, a trusted friend, or another guide. Sometimes what feels confusing to you in the moment becomes clear when you describe it to someone else. Remember: The fact that your guide has genuinely helped you doesn't mean they can't also harm you. Both can be true, which is why this work requires ongoing discernment rather than blind trust or loyalty.

⁂

Facilitating psychedelic healing work is akin to working with a live electrical wire. A guide, like a trained electrician, should be diligent and familiar with what is needed to keep everyone safe. Clearly stated boundaries help keep our feet on the ground of consensual reality and avoid the delusion that only oneness exists.

Currently, much of this work is happening in an underground culture without regulations or enforceable rules. In any group of people, some will be emotionally mature, have an inner moral compass, and be aware of the impact of their actions. Others will not. While an elder who has worked as a healer for decades may have years of hard-earned wisdom, they may not have a well-developed conscience. Unfortunately, this isn't about a few careless individuals. The absence of oversight, combined with clients who are eager for healing and don't know the red flags to watch for, creates conditions where sloppy behavior goes unchecked, and some of that sloppiness crosses into harm.

The work of finding a trustworthy guide requires self-awareness and a willingness to trust your instincts. You're being asked to stay alert and discerning while also being open and vulnerable. That tension is real, and navigating it is an ongoing practice, not something you can resolve once and for all. By understanding the dynamics explored in this chapter—power imbalances, amplification effects, projections, and boundaries—you're better equipped to recognize when something is off and to advocate for yourself or walk away.

The great majority of psychedelic guides are sincere, caring practitioners doing their best to facilitate healing, willing to learn from their mistakes and grow. However, I would be remiss not to acknowledge that some guides cross lines that go far beyond sloppy boundaries or unconscious dynamics. Your healing journey is too precious to leave solely in someone else's hands. Stay awake and remember that you are the ultimate authority on your own experience.

CHAPTER 11

Red Flags and Responding to Abuse

You have the right to safe, ethical care. Most guides and facilitators are caring, well-intentioned professionals, but not all maintain the same standards. The abuse of power that appears in psychedelic healing is not simply a matter of a few bad actors. It is a pattern that shows up across the field, just as it does in governance, religious institutions, education, and every professional arena. Wherever one person holds power over another's vulnerability, the conditions for misuse exist. Framing this as a problem of individuals lets the larger systems off the hook.

Part of ending the cycles of abuse is recognizing it for what it is, seeking support, and speaking out when appropriate. Harmful behavior needs to be confronted, and we need to take care of ourselves and one another when we encounter it.

You'll encounter psychedelic guides with eccentric styles and unconventional approaches; some of the most gifted healers don't fit conventional molds. The critical distinction is between practitioners who are simply unorthodox and those whose behavior is unethical or abusive. In an emerging field with few formal regulations, knowing this difference helps you trust your instincts and make informed decisions about your safety and healing.

This chapter is a reference guide to help you evaluate your guide's behavior if you are concerned about an interaction. I've divided concerning behaviors into two categories: orange flags, which suggest the need for questions and clarification, and red flags, which indicate serious violations that require immediate action.

Orange Flags

If your guide does any of the following, ask questions and seek clarity. They may be undertrained, lack sufficient boundaries, or need more supervision.

PUSHING AN AGENDA OR COERCION

- **Overpromises results**: There are limits to healing with psychedelics. If someone doesn't acknowledge this and evangelizes miraculous benefits, they're either new to the work or trying hard to sell you something.
- **Pressures you to take more medicine**: Sometimes it's appropriate for your guide to offer a booster, but this should be discussed beforehand. Taking more should always be your choice.
- **Pushes their personal agenda**: A guide's agenda about "where you need to go" can rob you of discovering things in your own way. Some people find an assertive style reassuring, but consider whether this crosses into controlling behavior.
- **Leads instead of follows**: From your first meeting, observe how well they follow your lead. They should listen intently, never putting words in your mouth or talking over you. Watch for all-knowing statements like, "You were definitely neglected as a child" as opposed to curious questions like, "Do you think the way your father treated you may have been neglectful?"
- **Encourages you to cut off relationships**: Unless they're supporting your own decision to end an unhealthy relationship, they shouldn't be directing your personal decisions.

- **Is not transparent and forthcoming**: You should feel comfortable asking about a guide's training, methods, approach to touch, and anything else that will affect your experience. If they're vague or avoidant, it's an orange flag. An ethical practitioner explains their methods clearly and acknowledges their limitations.

UNPREPARED OR OVEREXTENDED

- **Unprepared**: They arrive for your journey without having read your intake form, planned your dosage, or prepared a playlist.
- **Overextended**: Signs include disorganized scheduling, failing to take notes, leading a large group ceremony without enough support (a commonly recommended ratio is one facilitator or assistant per three to five participants), or neglecting preparation and integration support.
- **Sloppy**: The journey or ceremony space is dirty or poorly maintained. Rustic is fine; unsanitary is not.
- **Stressed or unwell**: If a guide is ill, scattered, or preoccupied with family matters requiring their attention, they should clear their schedule and prioritize self-care before facilitating. It's not responsible to accompany anyone into an expanded state without being internally prepared.

INATTENTIVE OR DISMISSIVE

- **Distracted**: They're on an electronic device during your journey (except to change the music). Phones, tablets, and laptops should otherwise be left in another room.
- **Negligent**: They leave the room before you're ready to be alone or don't offer you snacks and water at the end of a long journey.
- **Unresponsive to your requests**: They ignore your request to turn the music down, respond dismissively, or show hostility. A good guide is responsive and respectful.

- **Overshares**: Many guides share some personal information to build rapport, but when they reveal too much about their personal life and relationships, it shifts the focus from you to them.
- **Lack of humility**: If your guide seems overconfident or arrogant, be cautious. It's possible to be an effective healer while maintaining humility. The best guides tend to be down-to-earth.

POOR BOUNDARIES

- **Money and gifts**: A guide should be professional about the exchange of money, gifts, and time. When mistakes occur, they should discuss them openly and apologize when appropriate.
- **Mixing roles**: They shouldn't pursue any relationship with you outside the facilitator-participant dynamic. If they invite you to join another group or to become an assistant, you're moving toward a dual relationship that can muddy the therapeutic container. Any hint of romantic interest should be taken seriously and addressed immediately.
- **Inappropriate communication**: Guides should not extensively text or email about therapeutic material outside of scheduled sessions. Brief extra integration check-ins by phone or video are normal, but discussing therapeutic content at length via text or email is an orange flag.
- **Lack of supervision**: Both licensed and underground practitioners encounter ethical dilemmas and should have a network of professional support. Someone working in complete isolation is cause for concern.
- **Disregarding confidentiality**: They should keep every detail of their work with you private and should not share identifying details about other clients with you. If they talk about other clients with you, they are probably talking about you with them.

Most of these orange flags reflect undertrained guides, not malicious ones. Many concerns can be resolved through direct conversation. What follows is different.

Red Flags

If your facilitator does any of the following during a session or at any other time, demand that they stop immediately. You should seek support, report their behavior to their supervisor, and when necessary, contact a lawyer or the police.

TOUCH AND CONSENT VIOLATIONS

Your guide should never:

- **Touch your body without consent:** They need both prior agreement and permission in the moment. Exceptions include helping you to the bathroom or keeping you safe.
- **Pressure you to give consent for touch:** Consent should be freely given, never coerced. If you feel pressured at any point before or during the session, that's a violation.
- **Coerce you into receiving bodywork or energy work**: Any kind of bodywork or energy work should be clearly described beforehand and optional. If you ask them to stop, they should stop immediately.
- **Flirt or express sexual energy:** Any flirting or sexual energy from a facilitator is inappropriate. This includes suggestive comments or any behavior that feels sexualized.
- **Introduce full-body contact:** Cuddling or other full-body contact is inappropriate unless they have specialized training in a bodywork approach that includes this type of touch. Even then, you should have had a prior conversation with explicit consent, and they must still ask for your permission in the moment.

SEXUAL MISCONDUCT

Unless your facilitator has received specific training in a sexological modality and you have explicitly signed up for this service, your facilitator should never:

- **Encourage you to remove clothing** or remove their own clothing.
- **Kiss you** or touch your breasts or genitals.
- **Engage in any sexual contact** with you during the session, in integration sessions, or at any other time.

What If You Experience Abuse?

What can you do if your guide or facilitator has harmed you? First, get outside support. Reach out to friends or community members who will listen without judgment and validate your experience. Seek out a therapist or an organization that supports survivors of abuse.

HAVE A CONVERSATION IF YOU CAN

In unregulated settings, there is no formal complaint process. That said, you still have options. You can start by addressing your facilitator directly and asking them why they did what they did. You have no obligation to be forgiving or understanding; your only job is to be honest about your experience. There are genuine misunderstandings: a clumsy comment that landed badly, or something you misheard in an altered state. A direct conversation can sometimes clarify what happened.

However, if your facilitator blames your "sensitivities" or "trauma history" for your concerns rather than taking them seriously, that is a red flag. Trust yourself. If something felt wrong, it deserves to be addressed, regardless of whether it was intentional. Most unconscious behavior is unintentional. That doesn't make it okay.

If they become defensive, minimize what happened, or turn it back on you, that tells you everything you need to know.

A mature facilitator will approach reparative conversations with humility, taking full accountability for their actions. If they are able to take responsibility for any missteps, that's a good sign. However, it doesn't obligate you to continue working with them. Some violations irreparably damage trust, even with sincere apologies. You get to decide if repair is possible or desirable and whether you want to continue the relationship.

If a direct conversation doesn't resolve the issue, consider seeking an impartial mediator. If they aren't willing or able to join a mediated conversation, don't work with that person again. They don't have the relational skills necessary to offer this kind of work.

IN A CLINICAL SETTING

If you can point to negligent or unskillful behavior by a staff member in a regulated setting, you can start with a personal conversation or consider making a formal complaint. Whether or not it gets taken seriously depends on the clinic's leadership. Before signing up for a session at a private or corporate-run clinic, research the founders. Is the clinic run by experienced psychedelic guides and trained therapists? Or is it run by enthusiastic entrepreneurs serving a board of investors? Do they have established ethical guidelines?

GOING PUBLIC

If your facilitator's behavior is dangerous and they deny wrongdoing, you may want to share your experience more widely. Sharing your story, whether privately or publicly, is not about revenge or destroying someone's reputation. It's about protecting yourself and others and speaking your truth. If you want to make your experience public, it can be helpful to first consult a lawyer about potential risks and to work with a therapist or build a support circle as you prepare to do so. Public disclosure carries risks, including possible retaliation or legal threats, but it can also protect others. When no other accountability processes exist, speaking publicly can spark necessary community conversations and be part of your own healing.

If you've experienced abuse, be compassionate and treat yourself as you would treat a dear friend in the same situation. Healing from violation takes time, and there's no set timeline. You may feel confused, ashamed, or angry, all of which are normal responses. Take the space you need to process and heal. It isn't your fault.

What If You Witness Abuse?

What if you see something troubling happen to another participant during a ceremony? You have a responsibility to the person being harmed, even if they don't recognize the behavior as harm in the moment. If you are sober, able, and can safely intervene without escalating the situation, do so. If the situation is dangerous, trust your instincts and get help from fellow participants or assistants.

Document what you witnessed as soon as possible; write down details while they're fresh, including dates, times, and exactly what you saw. This documentation can be crucial if the person decides to report the incident later. Remember that your perception is altered in a non-ordinary state of consciousness, which can make it hard to trust what you think you saw, heard, or felt. That said, always err on the side of checking in rather than staying silent.

Check in with them privately. Share what you observed and ask how they're doing. They may not be ready to name what happened as a violation, and you shouldn't push it. Just let them know you're available if they want to talk. Try to be a compassionate witness, offer support, and be willing to speak up if asked. Sometimes survivors need time to think through what happened before they're ready to address it, and your willingness to validate their experience, whenever they're ready, can make all the difference.

We need to do more than expand our consciousness together. We need to listen to one another's stories, increase our self-awareness, and be sober, awake allies for one another.

CHAPTER 12

Remembering Our Way Home

Years ago I was at a book reading when I saw Ram Dass sitting in his wheelchair a few aisles over. Born Richard Alpert, he was the early psychedelic pioneer turned spiritual seeker turned spiritual teacher and elder. Though he'd experienced a near-fatal stroke and looked smaller, with a shock of bright-white hair, I recognized him immediately. After the reading, I waited until he was alone and walked over. I stepped forward and smiled. He looked up and smiled back, his blue eyes beaming.

"You don't know me," I started, "but I've known of you since I was young. I read *The Psychedelic Experience* and it changed my life. I went on to study dharma, train with healers, and devote myself to psychedelic healing." I took a breath, feeling a flush of pride. "Your book put me on this path, and I've dedicated my life to this work. I just wanted to let you know."

He looked at me, still smiling, and motioned me closer. I leaned in. He held my gaze for a moment, then whispered, "We are all doing the same work here."

A few seconds passed. Slowly, I nodded. I had wanted him to know we were in the same club; he wanted me to know there was no club. I thanked him and walked away.

The work takes countless forms. Raising a family, growing food, tending animals, making art, showing up for your community, going to therapy, and spiritual practice—all are ways people come to know themselves more honestly and open their hearts. Every human wants to feel fulfilled and loved, and will find creative ways to do so. Psychedelics are one path among many. Plenty of people live rich, awake, compassionate lives without these medicines, and using them confers no moral or spiritual superiority. There are many ways up the mountain.

And yet, life is hard, and there are times when we need to recover or restore ourselves. Psychedelics are medicine, in the truest sense of the word. Psilocybin is helping people with depression, with the symptoms of traumatic brain injury, and with end-of-life anxiety. Trauma survivors have watched their PTSD symptoms diminish after guided MDMA sessions, and ketamine is offering rapid relief from suicidal thoughts and chronic pain. People are using these medicines to break free from addiction and to seek vision when they are at a crossroads. Communities come together with psychedelic sacraments to share ceremony and prayer. These medicines are not a cure-all, but for many they are a turning point.

Perhaps unsurprisingly, pharmaceutical companies are trying to strip the consciousness-expanding effects out of these medicines so people can get the health benefits without the long hours and "mystical nonsense." But that "mystical nonsense" may be the deepest, most precious gift these medicines offer.

Once during a mushroom journey, I was sitting on a deck in a pine forest when a northern flicker, a stunning brown-and-black spotted woodpecker, visited me. She spent what seemed like an eternity foraging around in the leaves beside me as I watched her, mesmerized. Eventually she took flight and flashed me with her breathtaking scarlet underwing feathers. Her regal presence burrowed into my consciousness and has stayed with me for years.

The following spring I bought bird feeders and filled them with sunflower seeds, hoping to be graced by the flicker again. Was I a better person for having had that encounter? No. But my life felt richer. I remembered, just a little more, that I'm part of a greater living ecosystem that is mysterious and charming.

Psychedelic experiences can do that. They can shift us out of our self-absorbed lives and remind us that we belong to something larger, directing our attention to the grandeur of the living universe. They often remind us that we are threads in the tapestry of life, no better but also no worse than any other creature we share this planet with. They can be a remedy for the overwhelm and cynicism so many of us carry and remind us that humor, laughter, and compassion are subversive acts.

They can show us that life is a sacred gift.

And gifts come with responsibility. The earth gives forth so generously, yet many psychedelic medicines are limited and precious. When we receive something precious, it creates a small vacuum in the energetic field, what author Martín Prechtel calls a mutual indebtedness. To maintain balance, we traditionally give something in return. If we don't, nature rebalances in other ways, sometimes by taking something away. If you are fortunate enough to receive a gift from these medicines, consider giving back.

There are many ways to give back. You can join a local psychedelic integration group and show up to support others. You can volunteer with groups advocating for equitable drug policy and harm reduction. You can donate to Indigenous-led organizations working to keep their healing traditions alive. If you can, consider sponsoring psychedelic sessions for people who can't afford them by supporting clinics or healing centers that make services available to people from marginalized communities. If you feel safe doing so, share your personal experiences openly. You can give your time, your money, your skills, or your voice.

You can also give back by how you engage with your own path. When you ask thoughtful questions before choosing a psychedelic guide, you signal that diligence and integrity matter, and when you arrive at a ceremony prepared and aware, it raises the bar for everyone in the room. When you speak up about violations or unethical behavior, you may be protecting the next person. Expanding our consciousness often reveals how interconnected life is. That recognition should strengthen our responsibility to one another, not bypass it. The personal healing we seek is intimately connected to collective responsibility. What good is consciousness without conscience?

You may finish this book and feel ready to move forward. Perhaps you've decided to start with ketamine therapy and see where that goes. Maybe you'll travel to one of the states that have legalized psilocybin for a guided journey, or look for an ethical, well-trained guide closer to home. Or perhaps you'll join a ceremony with a plant-medicine church, apply to a clinical trial, or wait until psilocybin is legal in your state. Maybe you've realized that this isn't the right time, or that psychedelic healing isn't your path at all. Whatever you decide, you now have the knowledge to make your choice with open eyes. Whatever brought you to this book, I hope you found what you needed. But more than that, I hope you found your own capacity to know what you need. Trust that. And when you don't know, keep asking.

Whatever you choose, remember: We are all doing the same work here.

A Blessing for Your Way

May you be deconstructed by suffering and reconstituted by grace. May the parts of you that no longer serve you die a clean death, and may the gifts and beauty lying latent within you emerge into life. May you have a wide view of your path, a vast perspective to rest in when you feel constricted or lost.

May your healers and teachers be rich in conscience, alert, and compassionate. May you have all the support you need, inner and outer.

May you be fortified down into the marrow of your bones, every cell vibrating with vitality, connected to the field of power all around us and to the luminosity of space itself. May you be courageous, full of heart, bold, and alive.

May you slay your demons as well as your gods.

May you recognize your body as a portal into the expanse of sacred creation. May you breathe in the immensity of the sky, drink in the breeze, stand close to fire and absorb its warmth, walk barefoot on the earth and sink into her steady love, swim in waters and be cleansed.

May you know just what you need, and sing it out loud every day. May you find your way to deeper compassion and clearer wisdom, whatever your path.

May you remember you are a child—not just of the earth, but of the cosmos—growing through your suffering and being awakened to truth.

May your hands rest on your heart and feel it full and warm, thumping in sync with the heartbeat of life.

Additional Resources

Additional resources are kept up-to-date at PsychedelicSeekersGuide.com.

Appendix A: The Three Mirrors: A Psychedelic Readiness Self-Assessment

Created by Kristina Hunter, psychedelic educator and author of *The Psychedelic Seeker's Guide*

and

Julie Megler, MSN, board-certified Psychiatric Mental Health Nurse Practitioner, consultant, and educator on psychedelic-assisted therapies

Before entering the territory of psychedelic healing, take time to assess three areas of your life for safety and readiness. Psychedelics affect your body, your mind, and your emotional life simultaneously with an unusual intensity. They can surface buried memories, aggravate existing conditions, and cause upheaval that takes time to resolve. This is not something to rush into. The more honestly you assess where you are before you move forward, the safer and more beneficial your experience is likely to be.

The first mirror looks at your physical safety and readiness: Can your body safely navigate a psychedelic experience? Do you have medical risk factors that require evaluation first?

The second mirror looks at your psychiatric and psychological safety and readiness: Can your mind work with what emerges? Do you have the psychological stability and resilience to navigate intense emotional territory?

The third mirror looks at the readiness of your life circumstances and support systems: Do you have the stability and support to sustain a deep experience and integrate it into your life?

HOW TO TAKE THIS ASSESSMENT

This assessment takes twenty to thirty minutes. Answer the questions honestly; this is for you alone. Your answers will help you determine what timing, approach, and support you need. Serious medical or psychological conditions may require consultation with a health care provider before proceeding.

- Answer each section completely before moving on.
- Take as much time as you need for an honest reflection.
- Note which questions make you uncomfortable: This can be valuable information.
- If you're unsure about an answer, explore your uncertainty in writing.
- At the end of each mirror, pause to notice what you're feeling emotionally and in your body.

The First Mirror: Your Physical Safety and Readiness

MEDICAL HISTORY AND CONDITIONS

We recommend an annual physical examination for everyone. If you have not visited your primary care provider in the past year, start there.

Cardiovascular

- ☐ Do you have high blood pressure, either controlled or uncontrolled? Uncontrolled high blood pressure is when your blood pressure is over 140/90 at rest. Controlled is when you take medication to keep your blood pressure in a normal range.

- ☐ Do you have any heart conditions: arrhythmia, heart disease, or have you had a previous heart attack?
- ☐ Have you had a stroke, or are you at high risk for stroke?
- ☐ Has a parent or sibling been diagnosed with cardiovascular disease or had a cardiac event such as a heart attack or stroke before age fifty-five?

Neurological

- ☐ Do you have a seizure disorder or a history of seizures?
- ☐ Have you had a traumatic brain injury (TBI), including a concussion, in the last three to six months? Even if you feel fine now, we recommend waiting three to six months after a TBI before using any psychedelic other than ketamine.
- ☐ Do you have a traumatic brain injury that still affects you?
- ☐ Do you have any neurological conditions, including multiple sclerosis or Parkinson's?

Pregnancy and Reproductive

- ☐ Are you pregnant?
- ☐ Are you trying to become pregnant?
- ☐ Are you nursing?

Metabolic and Other Physical Conditions

- ☐ Do you have liver disease or impaired liver function?
- ☐ Do you have kidney disease or impaired kidney function?
- ☐ Do you have type 1 or type 2 diabetes?
- ☐ Do you have any autoimmune conditions?

- ☐ Do you struggle with an eating disorder, active or in recovery?
- ☐ Are you currently physically ill or recovering from an illness or injury?
- ☐ Do you have a sleep disorder or chronic insomnia?

If you checked any of these boxes or weren't sure whether or not to check them, contact a medical professional familiar with psychedelics. They can review your medical history and determine which psychedelics, if any, are safe for you. Do not proceed without medical consultation.

If you have a heart condition, consult with your cardiologist. If you have an autoimmune condition, discuss with your medical provider how it might interact with immune system activation during a psychedelic experience.

CURRENT MEDICATIONS

Check the box for any medications and supplements you are currently taking. All of these can interact with psychedelics:

- ☐ SSRIs: Prozac (fluoxetine), Zoloft (sertraline), Lexapro (escitalopram), Celexa (citalopram), Paxil (paroxetine), Luvox (fluvoxamine)
- ☐ SNRIs: Effexor (venlafaxine), Cymbalta (duloxetine), Pristiq (desvenlafaxine)
- ☐ NDRI: Wellbutrin (bupropion)
- ☐ MAOIs: Nardil (phenelzine), Parnate (tranylcypromine), Marplan (isocarboxazid), Emsam (selegiline)
- ☐ Miscellaneous antidepressants or anxiolytics: Remeron (mirtazapine), Desyrel (trazodone), Buspar (buspirone), Neurontin (gabapentin)
- ☐ TCAs: Elavil (amitriptyline), Pamelor (nortriptyline), Anafranil (clomipramine), Tofranil (imipramine), Norpramin (desipramine), Silenor (doxepin), Surmontil (trimipramine), Asendin (amoxapine)
- ☐ Antihistamines: Chlor-Trimeton (chlorpheniramine), Benadryl (diphenhydramine)

- ☐ Benzodiazepines: Xanax (alprazolam), Valium (diazepam), Klonopin (clonazepam), Ativan (lorazepam), Librium (chlordiazepoxide), Restoril (temazepam)
- ☐ Mood stabilizers: lithium, Lamictal (lamotrigine), Depakote (divalproex), Depakene (valproic acid), Tegretol (carbamazepine), Topamax (topiramate), Keppra (levetiracetam)
- ☐ First-generation antipsychotics: Haldol (haloperidol), Thorazine (chlorpromazine), Prolixin (fluphenazine), Trilafon (perphenazine), Loxitane (loxapine), Orap (pimozide), Mellaril (thioridazine), Navane (thiothixene)
- ☐ Second-generation antipsychotics: Abilify (aripiprazole), Clozaril (clozapine), Zyprexa (olanzapine), Seroquel (quetiapine), Risperdal (risperidone), Saphris (asenapine), Rexulti (brexpiprazole), Vraylar (cariprazine), Fanapt (iloperidone), Caplyta (lumateperone), Latuda (lurasidone), Invega (paliperidone), Geodon (ziprasidone)
- ☐ Stimulants: Adderall (mixed amphetamine salts), Ritalin (methylphenidate), Vyvanse (lisdexamfetamine), Dexedrine (dextroamphetamine)
- ☐ Weight-loss drugs: Ozempic or Wegovy (semaglutide), Zepbound (tirzepatide), Contrave (naltrexone and bupropion), Qsymia (phentermine and topiramate)
- ☐ St. John's wort or SAM-e
- ☐ Blood pressure medications
- ☐ Blood thinners
- ☐ Do you have any history of psychiatric medication use, including for sleep?

List other medications and supplements you are currently taking:

____

____

____

If you checked any of these boxes, including any history of psychiatric medication, consult a medical professional familiar with psychedelics. They can research specific interactions for the psychedelic medicine you're considering.

Some of the medications listed here have dangerous interactions with psychedelics, while others may be safe. Note that many psychiatric medications require gradual tapering over weeks or months. Never stop medications abruptly without medical supervision. This list is not exhaustive; if you are taking a medication that isn't listed and falls into any of the categories, consult a medical professional.

Critical Drug Interactions

- SSRIs and SNRIs can reduce or block the effects of some psychedelics, including MDMA, psilocybin, and LSD.
- MDMA combined with an MAOI or ayahuasca can be fatal due to serotonin syndrome.
- Stimulants combined with MDMA can cause dangerously high blood pressure and body temperature.
- Lithium or tramadol when combined with psychedelics can increase seizure risk.
- Weight-loss drugs can interfere with metabolism, leading to the delayed onset of some psychedelics' effects, which impacts dosing.
- Benzodiazepines can decrease the effects of ketamine.

AGE CONSIDERATIONS

How old are you?

- ☐ Under 25: Your brain is still developing. Proceed with extra caution, especially if you have a family history of mental health disorders such as psychosis, bipolar disorder, or schizophrenia.
- ☐ 25–65
- ☐ Over 65: You may need adjusted dosing and extra medical screening.

- ☐ Over 70: When did you last see a cardiologist? Have you had an EKG recently? We recommend that everyone age 70 or older have routine cardiovascular lab tests and an EKG within the past year.

SUBSTANCE USE

Current Substance Use Patterns

How often do you drink alcohol?

- ☐ I don't drink
- ☐ Occasionally (a few times per month)
- ☐ Regularly (a few times per week)
- ☐ Daily or near-daily
- ☐ I drink more than I want to

How often do you use sedatives such as opioids, benzodiazepines, or hypnotics?

- ☐ I don't use sedatives
- ☐ Occasionally (a few times per month)
- ☐ Regularly (a few times per week)
- ☐ Daily or near-daily
- ☐ I use more than I want to
- ☐ The sedatives I use are prescribed, and I take them as prescribed
- ☐ The sedatives I use are not prescribed, or I take them beyond the specified amount

How often do you use ADHD medications or stimulants?

- ☐ I don't use ADHD meds or stimulants
- ☐ Occasionally (a few times per month)
- ☐ Regularly (a few times per week)
- ☐ Daily or near-daily

- ☐ I use more than I want to
- ☐ The ADHD meds or stimulants I use are prescribed, and I take them as prescribed
- ☐ The ADHD meds or stimulants I use are not prescribed, or I take them beyond the specified amount

How often do you use cannabis?

- ☐ I don't use cannabis
- ☐ Occasionally (a few times per month)
- ☐ Regularly (a few times per week)
- ☐ Daily or near-daily
- ☐ I use more than I want to

Do you use any other drugs for fun or to function? Which ones and how often?

____

____

____

Recreational use of alcohol or sedatives combined with ketamine can cause respiratory distress and be fatal. People with a history of stimulant addiction should not use MDMA. Regular prescribed stimulant use may not be a problem, and many people with ADHD can safely use psychedelics while on their medication. However, it's best to take a one- to three-day break from stimulants before a journey, and stimulants should not be taken on the same day as psychedelics. If you use stimulants or sedatives daily, even if it's within the recommended and prescribed amount, we recommend consulting with a health care provider before proceeding.

Regular or daily use of alcohol or cannabis isn't necessarily a contraindication, but both substances can dampen psychedelic effects. Alternatively, cannabis can significantly intensify certain psychedelic experiences in unpredictable ways, at times triggering anxiety or paranoia. We recommend abstaining from both alcohol and cannabis for at least one week before a psychedelic experience and at least three days afterward.

Substance Use Disorder, as Defined by the DSM-5

A problematic pattern of substance use with clinically significant distress or impairment, with at least two of the following within a twelve-month period:

- Substance used in greater amounts or for longer than intended
- Persistent desire to use or unsuccessful efforts to control use
- Significant time spent obtaining, using, and recovering from substance use
- Strong desire to use the substance (craving)
- Substance use is impairing ability to fulfill school, work, or home life
- Continued use despite social and interpersonal problems
- Giving up social, job, or recreational activities
- Recurrent use in physically hazardous situations
- Continued use despite knowledge of a persistent or recurrent physical or psychological problem related to substance use

Substance Use History and Recovery

- ☐ I'm actively struggling with addiction to alcohol or other substances, and it's affecting my relationships, work, or ability to care for myself.
- ☐ I've had difficulty managing my substance use within the past five years.
- ☐ I've struggled with addiction in the past and haven't worked on it in a formal treatment or recovery program.

- ☐ I'm in early recovery, less than one year sober.
- ☐ I've been in stable recovery for one to five years.
- ☐ I've been in long-term recovery for over five years.
- ☐ I have no history of addiction or problematic substance use.

If you checked any of the first four boxes in this section, psychedelics pose significant risks for you right now. Talk to an addiction specialist or your sponsor first. If you are stable or in long-term recovery, still proceed with caution as different psychedelics may have higher risks for relapse, depending on your history. Some recovery communities view using psychedelics as relapse; others don't. Either way, you want to navigate this decision thoughtfully.

REFLECTING ON YOUR PHYSICAL SAFETY AND READINESS

Pause here. What did this mirror show you? Write three to five sentences about what you noticed:

____

____

____

____

Green: You Are Safe and Ready

- ✦ You have no significant medical conditions.
- ✦ You are not on contraindicated medications.
- ✦ You have no active substance issues.
- ✦ There are no age-related risk factors.

→ Proceed to the second mirror.

Yellow: You Are Close to Being Safe and Ready

- ✦ You have minor health conditions that can be monitored.

- ✦ You are on medications that need adjustment or discussion.
- ✦ Your substance use should be evaluated first.
    - ✦ Not all substance use disorders rule out psychedelic use. Some people may need to detox before using psychedelics. For others, psychedelics may be potent tools in looking more closely at how substances are impacting your life and provide the motivation required to change patterns.
- ✦ You are in an age range (over age 65) that may require extra care.

→ Medical consultation is essential before proceeding. With proper support you may be able to move forward.

Red: You Are Not Safe or Ready

- ✦ You have severe cardiovascular or neurological conditions.
- ✦ You are on medications with potentially dangerous interactions.
- ✦ You have an active addiction.
- ✦ You are pregnant or nursing.
    - ✦ If you are nursing and would like to move forward, reach out to a health care provider to discuss an alternate plan.

→ Do not proceed until you've addressed these issues. See "Alternatives to Psychedelics" later in this appendix.

The Second Mirror: Your Psychiatric and Psychological Safety and Readiness

MENTAL HEALTH HISTORY

Serious Mental Health Diagnoses

Have you been diagnosed with any of the following?

☐ Schizophrenia

- ☐ Schizoaffective disorder (a combination of schizophrenia and mood disorder symptoms)
- ☐ Bipolar I disorder
- ☐ Psychotic disorder
- ☐ Dissociative identity disorder (DID) or other specified dissociative disorder (OSDD)

Have you experienced:

- ☐ a psychotic episode: hallucinations or delusions when not using substances, as in seeing or hearing things that aren't there, or having beliefs disconnected from reality
- ☐ a manic episode in the last three years: distinct periods of two or more days of elevated or irritable mood with decreased need for sleep, racing thoughts, or risky behavior
- ☐ psychiatric hospitalization in the past year
- ☐ a suicide attempt in the last year

If you checked any boxes in this section, you're in the red zone. Psychedelics are not appropriate for you right now, with the possible exception of supervised ketamine treatment. The risk of triggering or escalating mania or psychotic symptoms is high. Talk to a psychiatrist who understands psychedelics before considering this path. There may be exceptions for people with bipolar I disorder who have proper support, but these must be evaluated on a case-by-case basis. Have you ever experienced:

- ☐ a manic episode
- ☐ diagnosis of bipolar II disorder
- ☐ psychiatric hospitalization at any point in your life
- ☐ a suicide attempt at any point in your life
- ☐ suicidal ideation: making a plan, imagining how you might do it
- ☐ diagnosis of a personality disorder

- ☐ strong emotional states related to feelings of abandonment, rejection, or mistrust of others
- ☐ losing yourself in relationships or abandoning your needs for others

Do you have a first-degree family history (parent or sibling) of:

- ☐ schizophrenia
- ☐ psychotic disorders
- ☐ bipolar I disorder

If you checked any of these boxes, you're in the yellow zone. Consult a psychiatric professional who understands psychedelics. They can take a detailed family history and can help determine your personal risk. Personality disorder diagnoses can be associated with challenging experiences in altered states of consciousness.

Genetic predisposition to bipolar and psychotic disorders sometimes does not fully emerge until your early thirties, so it's crucial to rule out any underlying risk. If you are under age thirty and have had a manic episode—even without a bipolar diagnosis—get a psychiatric evaluation before proceeding.

If you are over thirty and have experienced one or more manic episodes triggered by substance use, you are in the yellow zone. Medical evaluation is necessary.

Treatment and Hospitalization History

- ☐ I have a psychiatrist or a psychiatric nurse practitioner.
- ☐ I've tried medications, and they have helped me.
- ☐ I've tried medications, but they didn't help or had harmful side effects.
- ☐ I've discussed psychedelics with my prescriber.
- ☐ If you have been hospitalized at any time, including for treatment of an eating disorder or substance use, when was your most recent hospitalization? __________
- ☐ I've never had psychiatric treatment.

This information is useful when speaking with a potential facilitator or clinician. Your treatment history will help them understand what you've already tried, what's worked, and what hasn't. If you've been hospitalized, make sure to let a potential facilitator know. If you've never had psychiatric treatment, that's worth noting too, especially if you checked boxes in the Mental Health History section.

Suicide Risk Factors

Previous suicide attempt

History of depression and other mental illnesses

Serious illness, such as chronic pain

Impulsive or aggressive tendencies

Current or prior history of adverse childhood experiences

Sense of hopelessness

Violence, victimization, or perpetration

Criminal or legal problems

Job or financial problems or loss

Substance abuse

Warning Signs of Suicide Risk

Making plans for suicide

Looking for a way to access lethal means

Talking or posting about wanting to die

Talking about being a burden, feeling trapped, or in unbearable pain

Extreme mood swings, increased anger or rage, or expressing hopelessness

Being isolated

Increased anxiety

Increased substance use

Sleeping too little or too much

CURRENT MENTAL HEALTH STATUS

Emotional Stability

Right now, how would you describe your mental or emotional state? Rate 1 to 5, where 1 means this is a significant challenge, and 5 means this is not a concern:

My overall emotional stability: ___

My ability to handle difficult feelings: ___

My sense of safety in my life: ___

My connection to hope and meaning: ___

My feelings of loneliness or isolation: ___

My fear of abandonment: ___

My fear of rejection: ___

My mistrust of others: ___

Current Challenges

☐ I'm experiencing suicidal thoughts with an active plan or access to means.

If yes, seek immediate help. Do not proceed with psychedelics.

☐ I'm in active crisis: recent major trauma, loss, or life upheaval.

- ☐ I'm experiencing anxiety and it affects my daily functioning.
- ☐ I'm experiencing depression that makes it hard to function.
- ☐ I dissociate involuntarily. This includes frequently zoning out or feeling numb when in mild to moderately stressful situations.
- ☐ I'm emotionally volatile: intense mood swings, outbursts.
- ☐ I'm having difficulty managing family or work responsibilities.
- ☐ I'm struggling with basic self-care: cooking, eating, brushing teeth, showering, getting out of bed, or doing laundry.

Recent Major Life Changes

In the past six months:

- ☐ I've experienced the death of someone close to me.
- ☐ I've experienced a serious illness or injury, mine or a loved one's.
- ☐ I've experienced divorce or a major relationship ending.
- ☐ I've experienced job loss or significant career change.
- ☐ I've experienced a major move to a new city or home.
- ☐ I've experienced other notable upheavals: ___________________

If you're in crisis, checked several of the challenges listed here, or have experienced recent major life changes, this may not be the right time for a journey. If someone close to you has died recently, look for a practitioner trained in working with grief. Psychedelics can amplify whatever's present, including anxiety and overwhelm. Consider waiting until you're more stable.

TRAUMA HISTORY

NOTE *If you are unsure whether your childhood involved trauma or significant stress, we recommend you take the "Adverse Childhood Experiences (ACEs) Questionnaire for Adults." There are several versions online, including https://americanspcc.org/take-the-aces-quiz/.*

- ☐ No significant trauma.
- ☐ I've experienced a single traumatic incident: accident, assault, natural disaster, etc.
- ☐ I've experienced childhood neglect or emotional abuse.
- ☐ I've experienced childhood physical or sexual abuse.
- ☐ I've experienced developmental or attachment trauma in unstable early relationships.
- ☐ I've experienced combat or war trauma.
- ☐ I've experienced medical trauma.
- ☐ I am experiencing ongoing trauma: domestic violence, discrimination, etc.
- ☐ I've experienced complex trauma: multiple types of trauma over an extended time, including relational trauma.
- ☐ I've had a traumatic psychedelic experience.

If you have a trauma history:

- ☐ I have a PTSD or C-PTSD diagnosis.
- ☐ I dissociate when stressed or triggered.
- ☐ I've done significant trauma-focused therapy: EMDR, somatic experiencing, etc.
- ☐ I've been in therapy but never directly addressed my trauma history.

A trauma history doesn't disqualify you from using psychedelics, but it does affect how you should approach them. If you have significant unprocessed trauma and aren't already in therapy, start weekly sessions with a trauma-informed therapist if you can. Choose trauma-friendly medicines like ketamine or MDMA in a low to moderate dosage range rather than classic psychedelics. Look for a psychedelic guide with comprehensive trauma training and at least five years' experience. Group settings are not recommended unless there is ample support, including trauma-informed assistants. A self-guided approach is not advised.

Symptoms of Dissociation

Mild: A sense of daydreaming or feeling slightly disconnected from your body

Severe: Depersonalization and feeling detached from your thoughts, feelings, or body

Memory gaps: Inability to recall important personal information, especially after a traumatic event

Derealization: Feeling disconnected from your environment, as if it isn't real

PSYCHOLOGICAL RESILIENCE

Check the statements that feel true:

- ☐ I can generally handle difficult emotions without becoming reactive or overwhelmed.
- ☐ I have specific practices that help me regulate when stressed.
- ☐ I can ask for help when I need it.
- ☐ I've faced hard things before and come through them.
- ☐ I have some understanding of my psychological patterns.
- ☐ I'm willing to see uncomfortable truths about myself.
- ☐ I can tolerate ambiguity and not knowing.
- ☐ I trust that challenging experiences can lead to growth.

The more boxes you checked in this section, the better equipped you are to navigate the challenging moments that could arise during a psychedelic journey. If you checked fewer than four, consider building resilience through therapy or contemplative practices before exploring psychedelics.

YOUR RELATIONSHIP WITH CONTROL AND SURRENDER

These questions predict how you'll respond when your usual defenses soften. Rate yourself 1 to 5, where 1 is never, and 5 is always:

When things don't go as planned, I can adapt: ___

When I feel vulnerable, I can stay present: ___

When emotions get intense, I can ride them out: ___

When I'm not in control, I can trust the process: ___

Reflect on these scenarios:

The last time something uncomfortable happened that I couldn't stop:

☐ I rode it out with relative calm.

☐ I felt anxious but got through it.

☐ I panicked or shut down.

☐ I dissociated or left my body.

☐ I tried everything to regain control.

My pattern with surrendering to forces larger than myself is:

Write two or three sentences. Do you surrender easily? To what or to whom? Never? Only in specific settings?

____

____

____

____

The essential question:

Are you prepared for an experience you can't stop once it starts?

☐ Yes, and that actually feels liberating.

☐ Yes, though it makes me nervous.

- ☐ I'm not sure; I'd need excellent support.
- ☐ No, that terrifies me.

If you answered "that terrifies me" or recognize that you need to feel in control, a psychedelic experience is likely to challenge you. This is not necessarily bad, but you'll need excellent support and should start with shorter-acting medicines like ketamine rather than LSD. You may benefit from therapeutic work around control issues before your first psychedelic experience.

REFLECTING ON YOUR PSYCHIATRIC AND PSYCHOLOGICAL SAFETY AND READINESS

Pause here. What did this mirror show you? Write two or three sentences about what you noticed:

____

____

____

____

Green: You Are Safe and Ready

- ✦ You have no severe mental health contraindications.
- ✦ You are emotionally stable most of the time.
- ✦ You have cultivated self-awareness and resilience.
- ✦ You can tolerate the loss of control, even if you are nervous about it.
- ✦ You've addressed your trauma history, or you have trauma-informed support in place.

→ Proceed to the third mirror.

Yellow: You Are Close to Being Safe and Ready

- ✦ You have some mental health concerns, but they're manageable.
- ✦ You are emotionally stable though somewhat fragile.

- ✦ You don't like the idea of losing control, but you are willing to work with it.
- ✦ You have unprocessed trauma and need specific support.
- ✦ You're in active treatment with a supportive psychiatrist.

→ Extra support is essential. Consult with someone who can help you evaluate which psychedelics would be an appropriate fit for you at this particular time. Consider ketamine in a clinical setting with a substantial integration plan. Continue to the third mirror.

Red: You Are Not Safe or Ready

- ✦ You are dealing with active mental health issues.
- ✦ You are currently in crisis or feel emotionally unstable much of the time.
- ✦ You are not comfortable feeling out of control.
- ✦ You have manic or psychotic symptoms or suicidal ideation.
- ✦ You do not have ongoing support or active treatment in place.

→ Psychedelics are not appropriate for you at this time. Focus on stabilization first and consider the list of alternatives at the end of this assessment.

We've gathered substantial information so far. Consider pausing and returning to the final section after a break.

The Third Mirror: Your Life Circumstances and Support Systems

BASIC STABILITY AND SECURITY

Housing Stability

- ☐ I have stable, secure housing.
- ☐ My housing is somewhat stable.

- ☐ I feel physically safe where I live.
- ☐ I'm experiencing housing insecurity.
- ☐ I do not feel safe where I live.

Financial Stability

- ☐ I have a stable income or employment.
- ☐ My finances are somewhat stable but tight.
- ☐ I'm in a financial crisis.
- ☐ I can afford professional support if needed.
- ☐ I cannot afford professional support.

Current Major Stressors

- ☐ I am in the middle of a custody battle or legal proceedings.
- ☐ I have immigration-status concerns.
- ☐ I have a professional license at risk.
- ☐ I am on probation or parole with drug testing.
- ☐ I'm in an unhealthy or abusive romantic, family, or work relationship.
- ☐ There is a serious illness in my family requiring my care.
- ☐ Other: ________________

If you selected multiple boxes indicating instability or current stressors, this may not be the right time for a psychedelic journey. Psychedelics can amplify whatever is happening in your life, including chaos and insecurity. Without a foundation of relative stability, a journey can sometimes add to your stress rather than resolving it. Consider waiting until your circumstances stabilize, or start with lower-risk options such as ketamine therapy in a supervised supportive setting.

SUPPORT SYSTEMS AND RELATIONSHIPS

Emotional Support Network

- ☐ I have close friends who are familiar with psychedelics.
- ☐ I'm part of a supportive community or support group.
- ☐ I have family members who support my healing path.
- ☐ I'm in a stable, supportive romantic relationship.
- ☐ I'm currently in therapy. (For how long: _______)

Check all that apply about your support system:

- ☐ Some people would show up if I needed help.
- ☐ I feel comfortable being vulnerable with selected people.
- ☐ I have people who can offer me support without trying to fix me.
- ☐ I know how to ask for support when I need it.
- ☐ I have backup plans if my primary support isn't available.

Count your checks across both sets of questions:

- ☐ 7 or more: You have robust support.
- ☐ 4 to 6: You have adequate support that may need strengthening.
- ☐ 1 to 3: Your support is thin. Strengthen it before moving forward.
- ☐ 0: You are isolated. This is a red flag that must be addressed first.

Intimate and Family Relationships

Current relationship status:

- ☐ I am single and stable.
- ☐ I'm in a supportive partnership.
- ☐ I'm in a relationship with some tension or challenges.
- ☐ I'm in an unstable or unhealthy relationship.

- ☐ I recently ended a significant relationship.
- ☐ I'm going through a separation or divorce.

If you have a partner:

- ☐ My partner is supportive of my interest in psychedelic healing.
- ☐ My partner is neutral or uncertain about my interest.
- ☐ My partner is threatened or in opposition to my interest.
- ☐ My partner is unaware that I'm considering it.

Children:

- ☐ I do not have children.
- ☐ I have children and can get stable childcare.
- ☐ I have children, but childcare is challenging.
- ☐ I'm a single parent with minimal backup support.

Relationship instability or active conflict can add stress, complicating your integration. Disapproval from a partner or a family member can create difficult dynamics. If you are a single parent, you will need extra support and planning.

Therapeutic Support

- ☐ I have a therapist, and they are supportive of me seeking out a psychedelic journey.
- ☐ I have a therapist, but I don't plan to share my interest in a psychedelic experience with them.
- ☐ I have a therapist, and they disapprove of my interest in psychedelics.
- ☐ I'm not in therapy.

We recommend that everyone have a therapist, counselor, group, or other form of support to help integrate psychedelic experiences. If you have a therapist, we strongly recommend telling them about your plans. Psychedelic experiences have a strong effect on your psychological state, both during and after your journey, and intentional integration support helps you make sense of what emerges and apply insights to your life.

INTERNAL PREPARATION

Background Knowledge

How much do you know about psychedelics?

- ☐ I understand the risks, contraindications, and realistic outcomes of their use.
- ☐ I understand that set, setting, and dosage matter enormously.
- ☐ I understand what red flags look like in guides or facilitators.
- ☐ I've educated myself about legal considerations.
- ☐ I've researched different settings and approaches.
- ☐ I've identified potential guides or settings.
- ☐ I've read multiple books or substantial articles.
- ☐ I've talked to people with personal experience.
- ☐ I know the differences between substances: psilocybin versus LSD versus MDMA, etc.
- ☐ I understand the importance of preparation and integration.

If you didn't check one of the first five boxes, you need more preparation. Continue educating yourself. Your knowledge will help you stay safe.

Motivation and Intentions

Why are you considering psychedelics? Check all that apply.

- ☐ I've tried multiple therapeutic approaches with little to no success.
- ☐ I have a clear intention or an area I want to look into.
- ☐ I'm curious about consciousness and want to explore.

- ☐ I'm seeking a spiritual connection or a mystical experience.
- ☐ Someone recommended it, and it sounds interesting.
- ☐ I want to process specific trauma or grief.
- ☐ I'm seeking clarity on life decisions or direction.
- ☐ I feel stuck in patterns and want to break free.
- ☐ I'm desperate: I'll try anything at this point.
- ☐ I want to understand myself better.
- ☐ I'm seeking healing from a physical illness.
- ☐ I want to repair or improve my relationships.
- ☐ I want to spark my creativity.
- ☐ I'm drawn to it, but I can't fully articulate why.

Expectations and Commitment

- ☐ I hope this helps, but I'm not expecting miracles.
- ☐ I think this will cure my anxiety, depression, trauma, or addiction.
- ☐ I do not know what to expect, and that's okay.
- ☐ I'm expecting a spiritual experience.
- ☐ I'm willing to prepare and accept whatever experience I have.
- ☐ I want the medicine to do the work for me.
- ☐ I expect difficult moments, and I'm as prepared as I can be.
- ☐ I understand this is a process that unfolds over time, not a single event.
- ☐ I'm willing to do preparation and integration work.
- ☐ I just want to feel better. I don't care how.

Looking at your answers here, which of the following statements feel true?

- ☐ Desperation is my primary driver.
- ☐ I'm seeking escape rather than growth.

- ☐ I want to bypass doing my own work.
- ☐ I'm feeling pressure from others rather than an internal pull.
- ☐ I have curiosity alongside a specific intention.
- ☐ I have realistic expectations: I understand that psychedelics are not a magic bullet and they cannot do all the work for me.
- ☐ I'm willing to participate actively in my healing.
- ☐ I understand this is part of a larger healing path.

TIME AND SPACE FOR INTEGRATION

Integration Capacity

- ☐ I can take two or three days completely off around a journey.
- ☐ I can reduce my responsibilities for a week after.
- ☐ I have a private space where I can rest and integrate as needed.
- ☐ My schedule is flexible enough to accommodate unexpected needs.
- ☐ I'm willing to prioritize integration over other commitments.

If you checked fewer than three boxes, reconsider the timing. Integration time is what will allow your experience to become part of your life and minimize disruption.

ACCESS AND RESOURCES

What options are realistically available to you?

- ☐ I can access psilocybin in a regulated setting (Oregon or Colorado).
- ☐ I can access ketamine clinics.
- ☐ I can apply to participate in clinical trials.
- ☐ I have access to plant-medicine churches.
- ☐ I have connections to underground guides.
- ☐ I can travel to retreat centers abroad.

- ☐ I have financial resources for professional support ($1,000–5,000 or more).
- ☐ I need lower-cost or free options.
- ☐ I'm considering a sitter or self-guided approaches.

Legal considerations I'm aware of:

- ☐ I understand the legal status of psychedelics in my state of residence.
- ☐ I've considered the potential legal consequences of obtaining or using psychedelics. (This is especially relevant for people of color, immigrants, professionals with licenses, and parents in custody situations.)
- ☐ I've considered whether my employer requires drug testing.
- ☐ I'm willing to accept the legal risks involved.
- ☐ I'm not comfortable taking legal risks and need to pursue only legal options.

If you need free or low-cost options, you are limited to low-fee practitioners, community ceremonies, peer support, or a self-guided journey, which is higher-risk. Alternatively, you can wait and save money. Don't let urgency or desperation push you into a situation with higher risk than you are comfortable with.

REFLECTING ON YOUR LIFE CIRCUMSTANCES AND SUPPORT SYSTEMS

Pause here. What did this mirror show you? Write two or three sentences about what you noticed:

____

____

____

____

____

Green: Your Circumstances and Support Systems Are Strong

- You have stable housing and basic security.
- You have a robust support system.
- You have supportive relationships or are stable alone.
- You have a good knowledge of psychedelics.
- You have healthy motivations.
- You have time and space for integration.
- You have access to appropriate resources.
- You understand the legal considerations.

→ Continue to the final assessment.

Yellow: Your Circumstances and Support Systems Are Adequate

- Your circumstances are somewhat stable with some concerns.
- Your support is limited but adequate.
- You have some relationship challenges.
- You are still learning about psychedelics but are committed to continuing your education.
- You have mixed motivations and some desperation.
- You have limited access or resources.

→ You can proceed, but first strengthen your support system, start conservatively, or choose legally accessible options.

Red: Your Circumstances and Support Systems Need Attention

- You have unstable housing or finances.
- You need to work on building a support system.
- You are in an unsupportive or unsafe relationship.

- ✦ Desperation is part of your motivation.
- ✦ You don't have access to appropriate settings.

→ Psychedelics are not appropriate right now. Attend to your life circumstances first.

FINAL REFLECTION: THE GUT CHECK

After completing this assessment, sit quietly for a few minutes. Notice what you're feeling in your body right now:

- ☐ Excitement or nervousness
- ☐ Tension or dread
- ☐ Relaxation or relief

The small voice inside: What is it saying?

- ☐ "Yes, this feels right, even if it's scary."
- ☐ "I'm not ready for this yet but will be someday."
- ☐ "No, this isn't my path."
- ☐ "I'm trying to convince myself."
- ☐ Other: ______________________________

Write two or three sentences about how you feel about moving forward:

____

____

____

____

____

____

____

Trust what you notice. Choosing to move forward slowly is wise, and choosing not to pursue psychedelics now, or ever, is completely fine. All that matters is what's right for you right now.

Looking in All Three Mirrors: Your Overall Readiness

Now that you've looked in all three mirrors, what's your overall picture? Review your results:

First mirror (physical safety): green ___ yellow ___ red ___

Second mirror (psychological safety): green ___ yellow ___ red ___

Third mirror (life circumstances): green ___ yellow ___ red ___

ALL GREEN

If all three mirrors show green, you're as ready as someone can be for a psychedelic experience. You have:

- medical clearance
- psychological stability and self-awareness
- supportive life circumstances
- realistic motivation and expectations
- knowledge to make informed choices

Recommended approach:

- Therapeutic dosage may be appropriate for you with proper preparation.
- Work with a trained guide or in well-supported settings.
- Classic psychedelics like psilocybin or ayahuasca are options.
- Follow preparation and integration protocols.

Next steps:

- Continue reading this book.
- Choose your medicine and setting thoughtfully.
- Find an appropriate guide or support.
- Allow adequate preparation time, a minimum of four to six weeks.
- Schedule integration support.

TWO GREEN AND ONE YELLOW

If two mirrors show green and one shows yellow, you're ready but need extra attention in one area.

If your first mirror (physical safety) was yellow:

- Get medical consultation before moving forward.
- Choose medicines carefully and avoid contraindications.
- Start with a lower dose, sometimes called a threshold dose or minidose.
- Have medical support available.
- Consider ketamine as a gentler option.

If your second mirror (psychological safety) was yellow:

- Work with a trauma-informed practitioner.
- Don't go self-guided.
- Consider ketamine or MDMA, which are gentler for trauma.
- Allow more time for preparation.
- Multiple integration sessions are essential.
- Have mental health support in place.

If your third mirror (life circumstances and support systems) was yellow:

- If possible, wait until your circumstances stabilize.
- Choose legal, lower-risk options like ketamine clinics.
- Strengthen your support system before proceeding.
- Reduce other stressors if possible.
- Stick to conservative dosing.

Recommended approach:

- Start with a threshold dose. Build familiarity before going deeper.
- Choose shorter-acting medicines like ketamine or perhaps psilocybin rather than LSD.

- Choose a supportive setting over a self-guided experience.
- Schedule extra preparation and integration time.
- Set up clear emergency protocols.

TWO YELLOW OR ANY RED

If two or more mirrors showed yellow, or if any mirror showed red: The mirrors are showing you that now is not the time for a psychedelic experience. It may become appropriate later, or you may find that other healing paths serve you better. Psychedelic experiences need supportive conditions to be beneficial and minimize harm. What needs to happen first?

If red or yellow in the first mirror (physical safety):

- Seek a medical or psychiatric consultation.
- Stick to supervised medication adjustments.
- Address substance use issues.
- Wait until your physical health improves.

Timeline: Reassess in three to six months.

If red or yellow in the second mirror (psychological safety):

- Stabilize mental health: therapy, or consider a psychiatric evaluation, and possibly medication.
- Build emotional resilience.
- Address trauma with trauma-focused therapy.
- Work with control issues.
- Wait until your condition is more stable.

Timeline: Reassess in six to twelve months, possibly longer.

If red or yellow in the third mirror (life circumstances and support systems):

- Build a support system.
- Stabilize housing and finances.
- Address unsafe relationships.

- Complete education about psychedelics.
- Save money for appropriate support.

Timeline: Reassess in three to twelve months, depending on the issues.
Important: Having a yellow or red doesn't mean you'll never do this work. It means you need to prepare in other areas first.

Alternatives to Psychedelics

If this assessment showed you that psychedelics are not appropriate right now, consider other modalities that might serve you better. There are many pathways to healing. Even if you're in the green zone, you may find the following alternatives valuable as preparation or complementary practices:

For trauma: EMDR, somatic experiencing, sensorimotor psychotherapy, trauma-informed yoga, neurofeedback

For depression or anxiety: cognitive-behavioral therapy (CBT), acceptance and commitment therapy (ACT), psychodynamic therapy, medication, transcranial magnetic stimulation (TMS), Dynamic Neural Retraining System (DNRS), exercise programs, meditation, community support

For spiritual seeking: trauma-informed or beginner-friendly meditation retreats, contemplative practices, time in nature, ritual without substances, the study of philosophy or sacred texts, breathwork, device-free retreats

To access expanded states without psychedelics: drumming journeys, breathwork, hypnotherapy, meditation, dreamwork, active imagination

For stuck patterns: weekly therapy, twelve-step programs, life coaching, behavior change programs such as acceptance and commitment therapy (ACT)

For grief: grief groups, ritual and ceremony, therapy, creative expression, nature immersion

For meaning and purpose: volunteering, creative work, spiritual community, mentorship, philosophical study, continue building strong relationships

For physical healing: functional medicine, acupuncture, bodywork, Dynamic Neural Retraining System (DNRS), energy healing, dietary interventions

Resources for Next Steps

If you're proceeding with psychedelics:

Continue reading this book for detailed guidance.

Seek support from a guide, therapist, or community.

Give yourself enough preparation time.

Set up integration support in advance.

If you're not ready now:

Identify what needs to happen first.

Address health or mental health concerns.

Build support structures.

Explore alternatives listed earlier.

Set a timeline for reassessment.

Emergency Resources

If you're in crisis:

Suicide and Crisis Lifeline: call or text 988

Crisis Text Line: Text HOME to 741741

Fireside Project psychedelic peer support line: 623-473-7433

SAMHSA National Helpline for substance abuse and mental health: 800-662-4357

In Conclusion

Whatever this assessment revealed, you've shown care for yourself by slowing down to look clearly at where you are. While this assessment will give you valuable information, it isn't the final word on your readiness. You can discuss your results with a therapist or trusted friend and reassess as your circumstances change. Give yourself time before making any decisions.

This assessment is for educational purposes and doesn't replace medical or psychological evaluation by qualified professionals. If you have serious concerns flagged by this assessment, consult with appropriate health care providers before proceeding with psychedelic exploration.

Appendix B: Questions to Ask Before Choosing a Psychedelic Guide

Once you connect for a conversation, consider the following questions. The final sections contain questions specific to particular identities or experiences. This list is extensive, so choose the questions that are relevant to you.

Pay attention not just to what the guide says, but also how they respond to your questions. How do you feel during and after the conversation? Trust takes time to build, and acknowledging your intuitive responses is part of the process.

Initial Screening

Availability and logistics:

- What is your availability for sessions over the next few months?
- What are your fees and cancellation policy? Do you offer a sliding scale?

Core Questions

Background and approach:

- How did you come to offer this work?
- By whom, when, and how were you trained?

- What was the length of your training?
- How long have you been offering this work?
- How do you approach this work?
- How many guided psychedelic experiences have you had yourself?

Safety and screening:

- Will you do a medical screening? What is your intake process?
- Do you consult with a doctor or other medical provider?
- Under what circumstances would you decline to work with a client?
- How do you manage confidentiality?
- Are you willing to talk with my therapist before or after my journey?
- What is your protocol if I have a medical emergency during a session?
- What types of challenging experiences have you witnessed, and how did you handle them?

Substances and dosing:

- What substances do you work with and why?
- How do you determine the dosage for someone?
- Where do you source your medicines? (They may not share names for safety reasons, but can give you a general sense.)
- Do you test the purity and potency of each new batch?

Setting details:

- Where do your sessions take place? Their home, your home, or a dedicated space?
- Who else would be present during my session? Cofacilitator, assistant, pets, or other participants?
- Will you also take medicine during my journey?
- What will you be doing while I'm in my journey?
- What kind of music do you play, and are you open to adjusting it based on my preferences, including silence?

- Do you take notes? Will I receive a copy of them?
- Will you stay with me until I feel ready to leave? Or is there a time you would like me to leave by?

Consent and boundaries:

- How do you approach informed consent and touch in sessions?
- What types of interventions might you use during my journey? Touch, bodywork, energy work, music or singing?
- How do you think about power dynamics in this work?
- How would you respond if erotic feelings came up between you and a client?
- Do you have any expectations of me as a client?

Worldview and beliefs:

- Do you see psychedelic healing through a lens of mental health, trauma recovery, attachment work, spiritual healing, consciousness exploration, or some other way?
- Do you consider yourself religious, spiritual, or an atheist?
- Are you a licensed therapist, coach, or minister? If so, what does that mean to you?
- Are you a spiritual teacher or a shaman? If so, what does that mean to you?
- How do your beliefs affect the way you work with clients?
- Have you had a mystical experience during a journey? How did you integrate it?
- Do you believe in invisible forces, spirits, or guides?
- Will you set up energetic protection for me during my journey if needed?
- Can you point me toward a book or podcast that can help me understand your approach to this work?

Integration and follow-up:

- How many integration sessions do you recommend?
- How will you support me after my session and through my integration? Are there specific approaches you use?
- If buried memories of abuse came to the surface in my work with you, how would you support me?
- What happens if I need support outside of our scheduled integration sessions? Is there an additional cost for this?
- How long will you be available to support me if I'm having a hard time afterward?
- How will you determine if the work we are doing together is working for me?

Accountability:

- Are you being mentored or supervised by anyone?
- Have you ever had a misunderstanding or gotten into a conflict with a client? How did you handle it?
- Has anyone ever filed a complaint against you? (in licensed contexts)
- Have you ever had a romantic or sexual relationship with a former client?
- Do you provide a contact I can reach out to if I have concerns about our work together? (third-party accountability)

Questions Based on Your Identity or Experience

If you are a person of color, Indigenous, LGBTQIA+, or disabled:

- How have you educated yourself about racism and how it might show up in our dynamic?
- How have you educated yourself about LGBTQIA+ issues?

- Have you worked with disabled clients before? How do you approach accessibility, and how can you make my session comfortable?
- Can I bring a trusted companion or support person to my session?

If you are neurodivergent:

- Have you worked with neurodivergent clients before? How do you adapt your approach?
- How do you handle sensory sensitivities during a session (sound, light, touch, scents)?
- Are you familiar with how psychedelics may affect people with ADHD or autism differently?

If you are a trauma survivor, especially with PTSD or C-PTSD:

- What is your training in trauma-informed care?
- What is your training in working with different styles of attachment?
- What is your understanding of how trauma can show up during psychedelic experiences?
- How do you approach consent if I become nonverbal or dissociate during a session?

If you've experienced religious trauma:

- How do you work with people who have experienced harm in religious settings?
- Can you provide a nonreligious or secular approach if that's what I need?

If you've experienced a traumatic psychedelic experience:

- How can you help me prepare for our work together?

If you're an older adult, working with terminal illness, or at the end of your life:

- Have you worked with clients in my age range?
- What have you learned about the specific needs of older participants?

- Do you have experience working with grief and loss, retirement, and multigenerational family issues?

If you're living with a terminal illness or at the end of your life:

- What experience do you have working with people in my condition?
- Can I bring a caregiver with me?
- How will you adjust my dosage and the setting to support me?

After Your Conversation

Take time to reflect. What is your gut sense after the conversation? Did you feel heard, respected, and satisfied with their responses? Do you feel open and curious to proceed, or do you need another conversation?

If the guide was dismissive or defensive, that is important information. If anything raised a concern, trust it. If you can, consider interviewing a few other guides before committing. Finding a trustworthy practitioner you feel safe with is worth the effort.

Notes

INTRODUCTION

1 Leary et al., *Psychedelic Experience.*

CHAPTER 1
How Do Psychedelic Medicines Heal?

1 Anderson et al., "Psilocybin-Assisted Group Therapy"; Bader et al., "Investigating the Therapeutic Efficacy," 908.
2 Agnorelli et al., "Neuroplasticity and Psychedelics."
3 Nardou et al., "Psychedelics Reopen," 790.
4 Plummer et al., "Examining the Potential."
5 Grof, *Realms of the Human Unconscious*, 33.
6 Lad, *Ayurveda*; World Naturopathic Federation, "Naturopathic Principle."
7 Malone et al., "Individual Experiences," 256.
8 Griffiths et al., "Effects of Psilocybin," 12.
9 Griffiths et al., "Psilocybin Occasioned," 649.
10 Wasson et al., *Persephone's Quest.*
11 Malone et al., "Individual Experiences," 256.
12 Wolynn, *It Didn't Start with You*; Yehuda and Lehrner, "Intergenerational Transmission," 243.
13 "Psychedelic Trials," Blossom Analysis.

CHAPTER 2
Psychedelic Safety: What You Need to Know

1 Krebs and Johansen, "Psychedelics and Mental Health"; Honk et al., "Longitudinal Associations," 194.

2 Kopra et al., "Adverse Experiences," 965.

3 Henríquez-Hernández et al., "Hofmann vs. Paracelsus," 148.

4 "Drug Combinations," TripSit, accessed December 5, 2024, https://combo.tripsit.me.

5 "Drug Combinations," TripSit; "Psychoactive substance index," Psychonautwiki, updated July 13, 2025, https://psychonautwiki.org/wiki/Psychoactive_substance_index.

6 Kopra et al., "Adverse Experiences," 965; Darke et al., "Retrospective Study," 1645.

7 Maté and Maté, *Myth of Normal*, 20.

8 Hart, *Drug Use*, 85–108.

9 American Psychiatric Association, *Diagnostic and Statistical Manual*, 523.

10 Krebs and Johansen, "Psychedelics and Mental Health"; Johnson et al., "Abuse Potential," 143.

11 "Worldwide Psychedelic Laws Tracker," Psychedelic Alpha, 2025, https://psychedelicalpha.com/data/worldwide-psychedelic-laws.

12 Australian Government, Therapeutic Goods Administration, "Change to Classification of Psilocybin and MDMA to Enable Prescribing by Authorised Psychiatrists," media release, February 3, 2023, www.tga.gov.au/news/media-releases/change-classification-psilocybin-and-mdma-enable-prescribing-authorised-psychiatrists.

13 Government of Canada, Health Canada, "Notice to Stakeholders: Requests to the Special Access Program (SAP) Involving Psychedelic-Assisted Psychotherapy," Drug Product Announcements, February 27, 2023, www.canada.ca/en/health-canada/services/drugs-health-products/drug-products/announcements/requests-special-access-program-psychedelic-assisted-psychotherapy.

14 Csete, "From the Mountaintops," 5; Félix et al., "Going After the Addiction," 3; Quintas and Arana, "Decriminalization," 125.

15 "Psychedelic Legalization & Decriminalization Tracker," Psychedelic Alpha, 2025, https://psychedelicalpha.com/data/psychedelic-laws.

CHAPTER 3
Choosing Your Setting

1 Leary et al., *Psychedelic Experience*, 103.

2 Hartogsohn, "Constructing Drug Effects," 1.

3 Evans, "New Wave."
4 Kappel et al., "Ultimate Guide."
5 Oregon Health Authority, Public Health Division, "Oregon Psilocybin Services," June 2022, https://sharedsystems.dhsoha.state.or.us/DHSForms/Served/le4226.pdf.
6 "Psychedelic Trials," Blossom Analysis.

CHAPTER 4
Working with a Psychedelic Guide

1 Tedlock, *Woman in the Shaman's Body*, ch. 4; Winkelman, "Shamanism," 47.
2 Levin et al., "Therapeutic Alliance"; Kamilar-Britt et al., "Therapeutic Alliance," 101.
3 Johnson et al., "Human Hallucinogen Research," 503; Mithoefer et al., *Manual for MDMA-Assisted Psychotherapy*.

CHAPTER 5
Choosing Your Medicine

1 Crocq, "History of Cannabis," 223.
2 Guzmán et al., "Worldwide Geographical Distribution," 189.
3 Stamets, *Psilocybin Mushrooms*, 23–35.
4 Guzmán, "Hallucinogenic Mushrooms," 404.
5 Brudner et al., "Examining Mystical Experiences," 950.
6 Glass-Coffin, "Shamanism," 58; Sharon, "Sacred Sanpedro," 77.
7 Huachuma Collective, "Collective Statement."
8 Harvard Divinity School, "Native American Church"; National Congress of American Indians, "Calling on Federal."
9 Krystal et al., "Ketamine," 774.
10 Pan et al., "Suicidal Ideation," 327.
11 Hovda et al., "Systematic Review," 262.
12 Yang et al., "Efficacy and Safety"; Shannon and Geller, "MDMA for PTSD."
13 Holze et al., "Pharmacokinetics," 658.
14 Obrist, "Obrist Interviews LSD Inventor."
15 Torres, "Use of Psychoactive Plants," 198.
16 Oaklander, "Inside Ibogaine."

CHAPTER 6
Preparing for Your Journey

1 Beyer, *Singing to the Plants*, 324.

2 Aday et al., "Great Expectations," 1091.

3 Carreón, "Does Closing Your Eyes."

CHAPTER 7
Crafting Your Intention

1 Pronovost-Morgan, "Harnessing Placebo," 866.

CHAPTER 8
Navigating Your Psychedelic Journey

1 Grof, *Realms of the Human Unconscious*, ch. 4; Kangaslampi and Lietz, "Psychedelics," 2341.

CHAPTER 9
Integration in Your Hands

1 Bathje et al., "Psychedelic Integration."

CHAPTER 10
Navigating Power with a Psychedelic Guide

1 Herbert, *Chapterhouse*, 81.

2 Jung, *Dream Analysis*, 53.

3 Grof, *LSD Psychotherapy*.

4 Taylor, *Peer Consultation Groups*, 215.

5 Carhart-Harris et al., "LSD Enhances Suggestibility"; Dupuis, "Psychedelics."

6 Jung, "Psychology of the Transference," 170.

7 McLane et al., "Respecting Autonomy."

Bibliography

Aday, Jacob S., Boris D. Heifets, Steven D. Pratscher, Ellen Bradley, Raymond Rosen, and Joshua D. Woolley. "Great Expectations: Recommendations for Improving the Methodological Rigor of Psychedelic Clinical Trials." *Psychopharmacology* 239, no. 6 (2022): 1989–2010. https://doi.org/10.1007/s00213-022-06123-7.

Agnorelli, Claudio, Meg Spriggs, Kate Godfrey, et al. "Neuroplasticity and Psychedelics: A Comprehensive Examination of Classic and Non-Classic Compounds in Pre and Clinical Models." *Neuroscience & Biobehavioral Reviews* 172 (2025): 106132. https://doi.org/10.1016/j.neubiorev.2025.106132.

American Psychiatric Association. *Diagnostic and Statistical Manual of Mental Disorders*, Fifth Edition. American Psychiatric Association, 2013.

Anderson, Brian T., Alexander Danforth, Paul R. Daroff, et al. "Psilocybin-Assisted Group Therapy for Demoralized Older Long-Term AIDS Survivor Men: An Open-Label Safety and Feasibility Pilot Study." *EClinicalMedicine* 27 (2020): 100538. https://doi.org/10.1016/j.eclinm.2020.100538.

Bader, Husam, Husam Farraj, Joud Maghnam, and Yazan Abu Omar. "Investigating the Therapeutic Efficacy of Psilocybin in Advanced Cancer Patients: A Comprehensive Review and Meta-Analysis." *World Journal of Clinical Oncology* 15, no. 7 (2024): 908–19. https://doi.org/10.5306/wjco.v15.i7.908.

Bathje, Geoff J., Eric Majeski, and Mesphina Kudowor. "Psychedelic Integration: An Analysis of the Concept and Its Practice." *Frontiers in Psychology* 13 (2022): 824077. https://doi.org/10.3389/fpsyg.2022.824077.

Beyer, Stephan V. *Singing to the Plants: A Guide to Mestizo Shamanism in the Upper Amazon*. University of New Mexico Press, 2009.

Brudner, Ryan, Erica Kaczmarek, Marc G. Blainey, et al. "Examining Mystical Experiences as a Predictor of Psilocybin-Assisted Psychotherapy for Treatment-Resistant Depression." *Journal of Psychopharmacology* 39, no. 9 (2025): 950–60. https://doi.org/10.1177/02698811251346697.

Carhart-Harris, Robin L., Mendel Kaelen, Matthew George Whalley, Mark Bolstridge, Amanda Feilding, and David J. Nutt. "LSD Enhances Suggestibility in Healthy Volunteers." *Psychopharmacology* 232 (2015): 785–94. https://doi.org/10.1007/s00213-014-3714-z.

Carreón, Mary. "Does Closing Your Eyes Actually Make You Trip Harder?" *DoubleBlind Mag*, June 11, 2025. https://doubleblindmag.com/does-closing-your-eyes-actually-make-you-trip-harder.

Crocq, Marc-Antoine. "History of Cannabis and the Endocannabinoid System." *Dialogues in Clinical Neuroscience* 22, no. 3 (2020): 223–28. https://doi.org/10.31887/DCNS.2020.22.3/mcrocq.

Csete, Joanne. "From the Mountaintops: What the World Can Learn from Drug Policy Change in Switzerland." Open Society Foundations. 2010. www.opensocietyfoundations.org/uploads/0bf8bd55-64a5-4c3c-9548-2132524db48e/from-the-mountaintops-en-20160212.pdf.

Darke, Shane, Johan Duflou, Amy Peacock, Michael Farrell, Wayne Hall, and Julia Lappin. "A Retrospective Study of the Characteristics and Toxicology of Cases of Lysergic Acid Diethylamide (LSD)- and Psilocybin-Related Death in Australia." *Addiction* 119, no. 8 (2024): 1645–55. https://doi.org/10.1111/add.16518.

Dupuis, David. "Psychedelics as Tools for Belief Transmission. Set, Setting, Suggestibility, and Persuasion in the Ritual Use of Hallucinogens." *Frontiers in Psychology* 12 (2021): 730031. https://doi.org/10.3389/fpsyg.2021.730031.

Evans, Jules. "A New Wave of Legal Psychedelic Churches." *Ecstatic Integration* (blog). April 8, 2025. www.ecstaticintegration.org/p/a-new-wave-of-legal-psychedelic-churches.

Félix, Sónia, Pedro Portugal, and Ana Tavares. "Going After the Addiction, Not the Addicted: The Impact of Drug Decriminalization in Portugal." IZA Institute of Labor Economics. July 2017. https://docs.iza.org/dp10895.pdf.

Forte, Robert, editor. *Entheogens and the Future of Religion*. Council on Spiritual Practices, 1997.

Glass-Coffin, Bonnie. "Shamanism and San Pedro Through Time: Some Notes on the Archaeology, History, and Continued Use of an Entheogen in Northern Peru." *Anthropology of Consciousness* 21, no. 1 (2010): 58–82. https://doi.org/10.1111/j.1556-3537.2010.01021.x.

Griffiths, Roland R., Robert Jesse, William A. Richards, et al. "Effects of Psilocybin on Religious and Spiritual Attitudes and Behaviors in Clergy from Various Major World Religions." *Psychedelic Medicine* 2, no. 1 (2025): 12–25. https://doi.org/10.1089/psymed.2023.0044.

Griffiths, Roland R., Matthew W. Johnson, William A. Richards, Brian D. Richards, Una McCann, and Robert Jesse. "Psilocybin Occasioned Mystical-Type Experiences: Immediate and Persisting Dose-Related Effects." *Psychopharmacology* 218, no. 4 (2011): 649–65. https://doi.org/10.1007/s00213-011-2358-5.

Grof, Stanislav. *LSD Psychotherapy: The Healing Potential of Psychedelic Medicine*. 4th edition. Multidisciplinary Association for Psychedelic Studies, 2008.

Grof, Stanislav. *Realms of the Human Unconscious: Observations from LSD Research*. Viking Press, 1975.

Grof, Stanislav. *When the Impossible Happens: Adventures in Non-Ordinary Realities*. St. Martin's Essentials, 2006.

Guzmán, Gastón. "Hallucinogenic Mushrooms in Mexico: An Overview." *Economic Botany* 62, no. 3 (2008): 404–12. https://doi.org/10.1007/s12231-008-9033-8.

Guzmán, Gastón, John W. Allen, and Jochen Gartz. "A Worldwide Geographical Distribution of the Neurotropic Fungi, an Analysis and Discussion." *Annali del Museo Civico di Rovereto* 14 (1998): 189–280. https://doi.org/10.1615/IntJMedMushr.v7.i12.70.

Hart, Carl L. *Drug Use for Grown-Ups: Chasing Liberty in the Land of Fear*. Penguin, 2021.

Hartogsohn, Ido. "Constructing Drug Effects: A History of Set and Setting." *Drug Science, Policy and Law* 3 (2017): 1–17. https://doi.org/10.1177/2050324516683325.

Harvard Divinity School. "The Native American Church and the Sacrament of Peyote." YouTube video. October 4, 2021. https://youtu.be/r4q60Klygs8.

Henríquez-Hernández, Luis Alberto, Jaime Rojas-Hernández, Domingo J. Quintana-Hernández, and Lucas F. Borkel. "Hofmann vs. Paracelsus: Do Psychedelics Defy the Basics of Toxicology?—A Systematic Review of the Main Ergolamines, Simple Tryptamines, and Phenylethylamines." *Toxics* 11, no. 2 (2023): 148. https://doi.org/10.3390/toxics11020148.

Herbert, Frank. *Chapterhouse: Dune*. Putnam, 1985.

Holze, Friederike, Matthias E. Liechti, Nadia R. P. W. Hutten, et al. "Pharmacokinetics and Pharmacodynamics of Lysergic Acid Diethylamide Microdoses in Healthy Participants." *Clinical Pharmacology & Therapeutics* 109, no. 3 (2021): 658–66. https://doi.org/10.1002/cpt.2057.

Honk, Ludwig A., Cecilia U. D. Stenfors, Simon B. Goldberg, et al. "Longitudinal Associations Between Psychedelic Use and Psychotic Symptoms in the United States and the United Kingdom." *Journal of Affective Disorders* 351 (2024): 194–201. https://doi.org/10.1016/j.jad.2024.01.197.

Hovda, Nicholas, Winslow Gerrish, William Frizzell, and Ryan Shackelford. "A Systematic Review of the Incidence of Medical Serious Adverse Events in Sub-Anesthetic Ketamine Treatment of Psychiatric Disorders." *Journal of Affective Disorders* 345 (2024): 262–71. https://doi.org/10.1016/j.jad.2023.10.120.

Huachuma Collective. "Collective Statement from the Curanderos and Curanderas of North Peru on the State of Conservation of the San Pedro Cactus, Their Traditional Knowledge, and the Use of Wild San Pedro by Foreigners." Colectivo Huachuma, February 10, 2025. www.huachumacollective.org/_files/ugd/7cb3ef_0e5d8257bd8447b1a37b5e60a9824a44.pdf.

Johnson, Matthew W., Roland R. Griffiths, and Robert Jesse. "The Abuse Potential of Medical Psilocybin According to the 8 Factors of the Controlled Substances Act." *Neuropharmacology* 142 (2018): 143–66. https://doi.org/10.1016/j.neuropharm.2018.05.012.

Johnson, Matthew W., William A. Richards, and Roland R. Griffiths. "Human Hallucinogen Research: Guidelines for Safety." *Journal of Psychopharmacology* 22, no. 6 (2008): 503–8. https://doi.org/10.1177/0269881108093587.

Jung, Carl G. *Dream Analysis: Notes of the Seminar Given in 1928–1930*. Edited by William McGuire. Princeton University Press, 1984.

Jung, Carl G. "The Psychology of the Transference." In *The Collected Works of C. G. Jung: Volume 16. Practice of Psychotherapy*. 2nd edition. Princeton University Press, 1946.

Kamilar-Britt, Philip, Elana B. Gordis, and Mitch Earleywine. "The Therapeutic Alliance in Psychedelic-Assisted Psychotherapy." *Psychedelic Medicine* 1, no. 3 (2023): 101–12. https://doi.org/10.1089/psymed.2023.0020.

Kangaslampi, Samuli, and Morten Lietz. "Psychedelics and Autobiographical Memory—Six Open Questions." *Psychopharmacology* 242, no. 10 (2025): 2341–48. https://doi.org/10.1007/s00213-025-06771-5.

Kappel, Joshua, Juliana Todeschi, George Winfrey, and Will Denney. "The Ultimate Guide to Colorado's Natural Medicine Health Act (SB23-290 Psychedelic Law)." *Insights: Vicente LLP*. August 22, 2025. https://vicentellp.com/insights/ultimate-guide-to-sb23290-colorado-natural-medicine-psychedelics-regulation-and-legalization-bill.

Kopra, Emma I., Jason A Ferris, Adam R. Winstock, Allan H. Young, and James J. Rucker. "Adverse Experiences Resulting in Emergency Medical Treatment Seeking Following the Use of Magic Mushrooms." *Journal of Psychopharmacology* 36, no. 8 (2022): 965–73. https://doi.org/10.1177/02698811221084063.

Krebs, Teri S., and Pål-Ørjan Johansen. "Psychedelics and Mental Health: A Population Study." *PLOS One* 8, no. 8 (2013): e63972. https://doi.org/10.1371/journal.pone.0063972.

Krystal, John, Chadi G. Abdallah, Gerard Sanacora, Dennis S. Charney, and Ronald S. Duman. "Ketamine: A Paradigm Shift for Depression Research and Treatment." *Neuron* 101, no. 5 (2019): 774–78. https://doi.org/10.1016/j.neuron.2019.02.005.

Lad, Vasant. *Ayurveda: The Science of Self-Healing*. Lotus Press, 1985.

Leary, Timothy, Ralph Metzner, and Richard Alpert. *The Psychedelic Experience: A Manual Based on the Tibetan Book of the Dead*. University Books, 1964.

Levin, Adam W., Rafaelle Lancelotta, Nathan D. Sepeda, et al. "The Therapeutic Alliance Between Study Participants and Intervention Facilitators Is Associated with Acute Effects and Clinical Outcomes in a Psilocybin-Assisted Therapy Trial for Major Depressive Disorder." *PLOS One* 19, no. 3 (2024): e0300501. https://doi.org/10.1371/journal.pone.0300501.

Malone, Tara, Sarah E. Mennenga, Jeffrey Guss, et al. "Individual Experiences in Four Cancer Patients Following Psilocybin-Assisted Psychotherapy." *Frontiers in Pharmacology* 9 (2018): 256. https://doi.org/10.3389/fphar.2018.00256.

Maté, Gabor, and Daniel Maté. *The Myth of Normal: Trauma, Illness, and Healing in a Toxic Culture*. Avery, 2022.

McLane, Hannah, Courtney Hutchison, Daniel Wikler, Timothy Howell, and Emma Knighton. "Respecting Autonomy in Altered States: Navigating Ethical Quandaries in Psychedelic Therapy." *BMJ Medical Ethics Blog*, December 22, 2021. https://blogs.bmj.com/medical-ethics/2021/12/22/respecting-autonomy-in-altered-states-navigating-ethical-quandaries-in-psychedelic-therapy.

Mithoefer, Michael C., Annie Mithoefer, Lisa Jerome, et al. *A Manual for MDMA-Assisted Psychotherapy in the Treatment of Posttraumatic Stress Disorder*. Multidisciplinary Association for Psychedelic Studies, 2017. https://maps.org/wp-content/uploads/2022/05/MDMA-Assisted-Psychotherapy-Treatment-Manual-V8.1-22AUG2017.pdf.

Nardou, Romain, Edward Sawyer, Young Jun Song, et al. "Psychedelics Reopen the Social Reward Learning Critical Period." *Nature* 618, no. 7966 (2023): 790–98. https://doi.org/10.1038/s41586-023-06204-3.

National Congress of American Indians. "Calling on Federal, State, and Local Governments to Protect and Respect Peyote (*Lophophora williamsii*) and Its Byproducts." *Chacruna*. February 11, 2022. https://chacruna.net/national-congress-american-indians-resolution-protect-peyote.

Oaklander, Mandy. "Inside Ibogaine, One of the Most Promising and Perilous Psychedelics for Addiction." *Time*, April 5, 2021. https://time.com/5951772/ibogaine-drug-treatment-addiction.

Obrist, Hans Ulrich. "Hans Ulrich Obrist Interviews LSD Inventor Albert Hofmann." Interview, Art Basel, 2004. Reprinted May 29, 2024. www.artbasel.com/stories/hans-ulrich-obrist-albert-hofmann-lsd-art-basel-conversations-20-years?lang=en.

Pan, Yiheng, Maria P. Gorenflo, Pamela B. Davis, David C. Kaelber, Susan De Luca, and Rong Xu. "Suicidal Ideation Following Ketamine Prescription in Patients with Recurrent Major Depressive Disorder: A Nation-Wide Cohort Study." *Translational Psychiatry* 14, no. 1 (2024): 327. https://doi.org/10.1038/s41398-024-03033-4.

Plummer, Zoe, Josh Allen, Justin Brand, Leah M. Mayo, Sandy R. Shultz, and Brian R. Christie. "Examining the Potential of Psilocybin and 5-MeO-DMT as Therapeutics for Traumatic Brain Injury." *Progress in Neuro-Psychopharmacology and Biological Psychiatry* 141 (2025): 111448. https://doi.org/10.1016/j.pnpbp.2025.111448.

Pollan, Michael. *How to Change Your Mind: What the New Science of Psychedelics Teaches Us About Consciousness, Dying, Addiction, Depression, and Transcendence*. Penguin, 2018.

Pronovost-Morgan, Chloé, Ido Hartogsohn, and Johannes G. Ramaekers. "Harnessing Placebo: Lessons from Psychedelic Science." *Journal of Psychopharmacology* 37, no. 9 (2023): 866–75. https://doi.org/10.1177/02698811231182602.

"Psychedelic Trials." Blossom Analysis. Accessed December 5, 2024. https://blossomanalysis.com/trials.

Quintas, Jorge, and Xabier Arana. "Decriminalization: Different Models in Portugal and Spain." In *Dual Markets: Comparative Approaches to Regulation*, edited by Francesco Calderoni, Mark Kleiman, and Ernesto Ugo Savona. Springer, 2017.

Shannon, Scott, and Jamarie Geller. "MDMA for PTSD and Beyond: A New Paradigm Brings Hope." *Frontiers in Human Neuroscience* 18 (2024): 1475013. https://doi.org/10.3389/fnhum.2024.1475013.

Sharon, Douglas. "Sacred Sanpedro in Ethnoarchaeological Context." *Ñawpa Pacha* 39, no. 1 (2019): 77–120. https://doi.org/10.1080/00776297.2019.1574959.

Stamets, Paul. *Psilocybin Mushrooms in Their Natural Habitats: A Guide to the History, Identification, and Use of Psychoactive Fungi*. Ten Speed Press, 2025.

Taylor, Kylea. *The Ethics of Caring: Finding Right Relationship with Clients*. Hanford Mead, 2017.

Taylor, Kylea. *Peer Consultation Groups & Ethical Awareness Tools for Psychedelic Practitioners*. Hanford Mead, 2024.

Tedlock, Barbara. *The Woman in the Shaman's Body: Reclaiming the Feminine in Religion and Medicine*. Random House, 2005.

Torres, Constantino Manuel. "The Use of Psychoactive Plants by Ancient Indigenous Populations of the North Andes." *Journal of Psychedelic Studies* 3, no. 2 (2019): 198–211. https://doi.org/10.1556/2054.2018.015.

Wasson, R. Gordon, Stella Kramrisch, Jonathan Ott, and Carl A. P. Ruck. *Persephone's Quest: Entheogens and the Origins of Religion*. Yale University Press, 1986.

Winkelman, Michael. "Shamanism in Cross-Cultural Perspective." *International Journal of Transpersonal Studies* 31, no. 2 (2012): 47–62. http://dx.doi.org/10.24972/ijts.2012.31.2.47.

Wolynn, Mark. *It Didn't Start with You: How Inherited Family Trauma Shapes Who We Are and How to End the Cycle*. Penguin Life, 2017.

World Naturopathic Federation. “Naturopathic Principle: Healing Power of Nature (Vis Medicatrix Naturae).” 2024. https://worldnaturopathicfederation.org/wp-content/uploads/2024/05/Healing-Power-of-Nature.pdf.

Yang, Jianhua, Ni Wang, Wulin Luo, and Junwei Gao. “The Efficacy and Safety of MDMA-Assisted Psychotherapy for Treatment of Posttraumatic Stress Disorder: A Systematic Review and Meta-Analysis from Randomized Controlled Trials.” *Psychiatry Research* 339 (2024): 116043. https://doi.org/10.1016/j.psychres.2024.116043.

Yehuda, Rachel, and Amy Lehrner. “Intergenerational Transmission of Trauma Effects: Putative Role of Epigenetic Mechanisms.” *World Psychiatry* 17, no. 3 (2018): 243–57. https://doi.org/10.1002/wps.20568.

Index

B

C

D

H

I

M

O

P

Q

R

S

U

V

W

Acknowledgments

A deep bow to Jed Fox, who brought his unwavering love and brilliant eye to every page of this book. He cooked the meals, walked the dogs, stoked the fires, keeping our world turning so I could dive into my writing.

Natalie Ostrowski, my sister, has been a steady force of goodness and sanity, reading chapter drafts and lifting my spirits. My mom, Rosalind Hunter, who instilled in me a zest for life and read a chapter anytime I asked. My father, Joseph Hunter, has been a gentle protector and encouraged me to take things apart and see how they work. And Ryan Hunter, Jasmine and Aila Bell, Daniel "the espresso master" Ostrowski, sweet Oliver James, and Mimi and Richard Fox: thank you for being good family. And countless treat balls of gratitude to my furry familiars, Nyima and Kunga, for getting me outside and making me laugh.

Thank you Tim McKee, Francesca Walker, Janelle Ludowise, Christopher Church, and the team at North Atlantic Books who gave this book a home. Andy Couturier, my writing mentor extraordinaire, who cheerleads me lovingly and teaches me how delightfully mystical writing can be. Bridget Lyons, a ferocious super-editor, returned drafts faster than humanly possible and brought her care and thoughtful suggestions to every page.

David Luce, my big brother on this zigzag path, read drafts, encouraged me relentlessly, and always answers the phone. Moana Meadow read every page with a rigor that is maddening and irreplaceable. Chloe Lieberman, my heart companion, shared soulful insights that made this a better book.

Thank you to Julie Megler, who brought her clinical precision and deep care to our Psychedelic Readiness Self-Assessment. Isaac Meadow's heartfelt conversations with me helped shape this book.

Raquel Bennett, the real "Ketamine Queen," for her psychedelic genius and encouragement over the years. Marisa Morin helped me dream this book into existence. I am grateful to my friends and colleagues who read sections of this book and helped me improve them: Zoe Benoît, Bear Begelman, Leon Segal, Brook Stone, Nancy Rhine, Erica Geller, Heather Findlay, Angella Okawa, Lindsay Branham, and Mieze Steinberg.

Thank you to my godfather and super mensch, Jack Lieberman, for his tremendous encouragement and generosity. He asked me to stay on the bus, and I stayed. Peter Young's kind support gave me the freedom to devote focused time to this book.

To my teachers on the San Juan Ridge: thank you for tending the mysteries and for dedicating your lives to soulful, conscientious transformation. Jo Wunderly gave me quiet, beautiful places to hide from the world and get some writing done. Michael Katz has shared gems with me over the years, from his decades of publishing wisdom.

Hank Snavely: I stole two of your books when I was twelve. I'm sorry about that, and thank you. They changed my life.

Thank you to Jennifer Shayna Gordon for teaching me how to draw the essence from the marrow. Jonathan Tenney, for being my guide and teacher for all these years. Lama Drimed, for teaching me to let my soul love what it loves. And Jennifer Welwood, for her effortless poetic incantations of awakening.

To my colleagues at the UC Berkeley Psychedelic Facilitation Certificate Program: Tina Trujillo, Moana Meadow, Susana Bustos, Kylea Taylor, Mary Sanders, Sylver Quevedo, Joseph Zamaria, Angella Okawa, Eve Ekman, Lindsay Branham, Joody Marks, and Christina Lacey. Three years of working alongside you all have made me a better thinker and practitioner. And to the three cohorts of graduates of the Certificate Program, thank you for your commitment to doing this work with integrity and for what we shared.

To the doctors, healers, and medicine carriers who have taken me under your care over the years, I would not be here without you. Thank you to the friends and neighbors in Martinez, California, who rallied around me and raised me up during my cancer recovery in 2012. I will never forget what you did.

I am grateful to all those I have the honor of working with, who trust me, teach me, call me out, and call me in. And to my dear friends and sangha brothers and sisters, for walking this sacred path with me.

To the healing plants and extraordinary molecules who have guided me, healed me, and shown me the way, thank you for your fierce love and infinite compassion.

I thank the truth tellers, the disrupters, the writers, the researchers, the lawyers, the activists, the journalists, the teachers, the guides, the ceremonialists, the community organizers, and everyone who takes risks to share good medicine, fights for cognitive liberty, and holds the line on relational integrity.

And to all those I have walked beside and learned from until our paths diverged.

This book wouldn't be, without you all.

About the Author

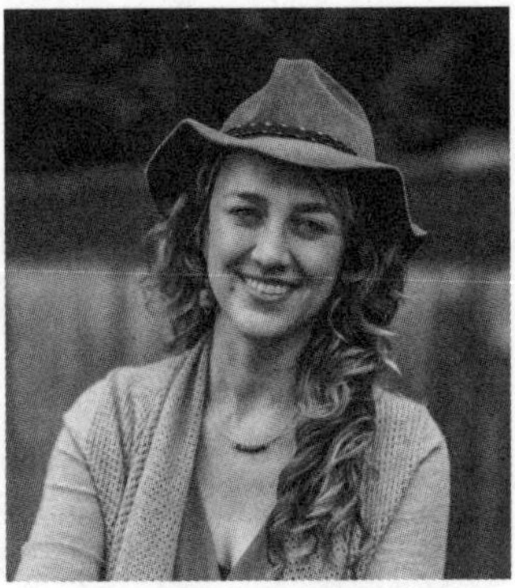

Photo credit: Jeff Leland

Kristina Hunter is a psychedelic educator and integration specialist based in Northern California and the coauthor of *Consciousness Medicine* (North Atlantic Books, 2019). She taught in the University of California, Berkeley's Psychedelic Facilitation Certificate Program from 2022 to 2025, training three cohorts of professionals in ethics and facilitation practices. A certified Hakomi mindfulness-based somatic counselor and a lifelong Buddhist practitioner with fifteen years of study and practice in the Vajrayana tradition, she has trained with medicine carriers and psychedelic guides in South America and the United States for more than twenty years. Kristina maintains a private psychedelic integration practice working with both newcomers and experienced practitioners and consults with clinicians on psychedelic facilitation, ethics, and harm reduction.

Kristina can be reached at https://kristinahunter.com.

About North Atlantic Books

North Atlantic Books (NAB) is an independent, nonprofit publisher committed to a bold exploration of the relationships between mind, body, spirit, and nature. Founded in 1974, NAB aims to nurture a holistic view of the arts, sciences, humanities, and healing. To make a donation or to learn more about our books, authors, events, and newsletter, please visit www.northatlanticbooks.com.